MCQ

Medical Library

Queen's University Belfast
Tel: 028 9063 2500
E-mail: med.issue@qub.ac.uk

For due dates and renewals:

QUB borrowers see 'MY ACCOUNT' at
http://library.qub.ac.uk/qcat
or go to the Library Home Page

HPSS borrowers see 'MY ACCOUNT' at
www.honni.qub.ac.uk/qcat

This book must be returned not later
than its due date but may be recalled
earlier if in demand

Fines are imposed on overdue books

Other books by F G Smiddy, published by Churchill Livingstone:

Smiddy F G *Tutorials in Clinical Surgery Volume 1*
Smiddy F G *Tutorials in Clinical Surgery Volume 2*
Cowen P N and Smiddy F G *Pocket Examiner in Pathology*

For Churchill Livingstone

Publisher: Timothy Horne
Project Editor: Janice Urquhart
Copy Editor: Alison Nicoll
Project Controller: Nancy Arnott
Design Direction: Erik Bigland

MCQs in General Pathology

F. G. Smiddy
MD ChM, FRCS
Former Consultant Surgeon, The General Infirmary at Leeds and Clayton Hospital, Wakefield; Former Senior Lecturer in Surgery, University of Leeds; Member of the Court of Examiners, the Royal College of Surgeons of England; Examiner in Pathology, Royal College of Surgeons of England.

J. L. Turk
MD DSC (London) FRCP FRCS FRCPath
Emeritus Sir William Collins Professor of Human and Comparative Pathology, the Royal College of Surgeons of England and the University of London; Examiner in Pathology, Royal College of Surgeons of England; Curator of the Hunterian Museum.

SECOND EDITION

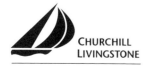
CHURCHILL
LIVINGSTONE

NEW YORK EDINBURGH LONDON MADRID MELBOURNE SAN FRANCISCO TOKYO 1997

CHURCHILL LIVINGSTONE
Medical Division of Pearson Professional Limited

Distributed in the United States of America by Churchill Livingstone Inc.,
650 Avenue of the Americas, New York, N.Y. 10011, and by associated
companies, branches and representatives throughout the world.

First published 1981 (Pitman Publishing Ltd)
Second edition 1997

ISBN 0 443 05419 3

British Library Cataloguing in Publication Data
A catalogue record for this book is available from the British Library

Library of Congress Cataloging in Publication Data
A catalog record for this book is available from the Library of Congress

Medical knowledge is constantly changing. As new information becomes
available, changes in treatment, procedures, equipment and the use of drugs
become necessary. The authors and the publishers have, as far as it is
possible, taken care to ensure that the information given in the text is accurate
and up to date. However, readers are strongly advised to confirm that the
information, especially with regard to drug usage, complies with current
legislation and standards of practice.

The
publisher's
policy is to use
**paper manufactured
from sustainable forests**

Produced by Longman Singapore Publishers (Pte) Ltd.
Printed in Singapore

Contents

Authors' Foreword

The object of this textbook is twofold. Firstly, many candidates in surgical and pathological examinations are faced with the problem of answering multiple choice questions and may wish to test both their knowledge and technique. They may also wish to time themselves against the clock in order to ascertain that their 'work rate' is satisfactory. In order to achieve this object, we have constructed over 300 questions governing the principles of general pathology and arranged the questions in groups of 20 questions in random fashion.

Secondly, a candidate may wish not only to practise the technique of answering the multiple choice question papers, but also to add to his knowledge. For this latter reason, in the second part of the book, each answer, whether it be true or false, is accompanied by an explanation.

The stimulus to write this book comes from our many years of examining candidates in General Pathology. Although it would be incorrect to suggest that this text is a substitute for a normal textbook, by dividing the questions into a variety of important topics, we have done our best to achieve a comprehensive cover of the subjects as a whole.

F. G. Smiddy
J. L. Turk

Preface

The authors of this book have been stimulated to write it following our contact with innumerable candidates in the Primary Fellowships of the various Royal Colleges. Although a radical change is occurring in the present fellowship examination with a division into the MRCS followed later by the specialist Fellowships, general pathology will continue to figure prominently in both examinations hence the continuing need for knowledge in this subject.

However not only candidates for higher surgical training require a knowledge of general pathology. We feel that the information contained in this short book will also assist the undergraduate student. Those candidates who wish to use this book solely for self assessment will find the questions in the first section have been arranged in random fashion and the correct answers, either true or false, have been indicated at the end of each paper.

In the second section the questions are repeated, but explanation is given as to the reason for the answers be they true or false. Thus the text forms not only a test of knowledge but also serves for revision of this subject.

F. G. S.
J. L. T.

Acknowledgements

It is with deep gratitude that the Authors acknowledge the great help given to them by Margaret Smith and Lynn Topham, our respective secretaries, who deal with many aspects of the unfinished manuscript.

It would also be right and proper to acknowledge the stimulus which the examination of numerous candidates in the Primary Fellowship gave us.

Part 1: Random questions

Each group of 20 questions is followed by the answers.

23.1 The chief effector cells involved in the rejection of a renal allograft are:
1. CD4+ T cells
2. CD8+ T cells
3. passenger leucocytes
4. platelets
5. B lymphocytes

7.24 Cell-mediated immunity involves the following mechanisms:
1. IgG
2. T lymphocytes
3. eosinophils
4. complement
5. macrophages

16.1 The chief pathological changes of atherosclerosis are:
1. deposition of lipid in the smooth muscle cells of the intima
2. fragmentation of the internal elastic lamina
3. calcification
4. contraction of the vessel
5. collagen deposition

10.3 Pulmonary oedema may occur in patients suffering from:
1. major trauma
2. plague
3. right-sided heart failure
4. hypoproteinaemia
5. nematode infections

1.3 Old age is specifically associated with atrophic changes in:
1. bone
2. the kidneys
3. the bone marrow
4. the brain
5. the ovaries

14.14 The following tumours may produce hormones:
1. choriocarcinoma
2. bronchial carcinoma
3. fibroma of the ovary
4. islet cell tumours of the pancreas
5. chromophobe pituitary adenoma

16.4 Gangrene is necrosis together with:
1. desiccation
2. colliquative necrosis
3. involvement of a limb
4. infection of the tissues with Gram-positive organisms
5. putrefaction

20.8 Hyperkalaemia commonly occurs:
1. following severe burns
2. in Conn's syndrome
3. following glomerular necrosis
4. in the Zollinger–Ellison syndrome
5. in the carcinoid syndrome

21.1 Blood which is to be used for transfusion:
1. should be stored at –4°C
2. may need to be irradiated (1000r)
3. needs to be tested for complement content
4. may be used after storage for platelet replacement
5. should be stored in an acid anticoagulant

3.5 Hyperplasia of the lymphoid tissue is a prominent feature in the following conditions:
1. toxoplasmosis
2. leishmaniasis
3. chronic dermatitis
4. silicosis
5. berylliosis

4.7 Pseudomembranous enterocolitis is caused by the following organisms:
1. *Clostridium sporogenes*
2. *Clostridium difficile*
3. *Streptococcus faecalis*
4. penicillin resistant staphylococci
5. *Pseudomonas aeruginosa*

4.5 The virulence of bacteria is related to:
1. their number in the tissues
2. the production of toxins
3. their ability to produce spreading factors
4. their resistance to phagocytosis
5. decreased resistance of the host

24.7   **The following are mainly intracellular parasites:**
1. *Echinococcus granulosus*
2. *Leishmania donovani*
3. *Trypanosoma gambiense*
4. *Plasmodium vivax*
5. *Toxoplasma gondii*

3.11   **The following metals cause epithelioid cell granulomas:**
1. beryllium
2. chromium
3. zirconium
4. nickel
5. iron

6.2   **The healing of an incised wound is associated with the following:**
1. a lag phase
2. a demolition phase
3. a proliferative phase
4. a contractile phase
5. a maturation phase

17.18   **Chronic myeloid leukaemia is associated with:**
1. the presence of large numbers of myeloblasts in the peripheral blood
2. a very variable total white count
3. massive splenomegaly
4. lymph node enlargement
5. hepatomegaly

18.7   **The plasma acid phosphatase concentration increases in:**
1. Paget's disease (osteitis deformans)
2. idiopathic hypercalciuria
3. prostatic cancer
4. medullary carcinoma of the thyroid
5. rickets

7.16   **Anaphylaxis:**
1. develops 24 hours after the initial stimulus
2. causes a weal and flare response
3. is produced by IgA antibody
4. causes eosinophilia
5. causes degranulation of basophils and mast cells

7.33   **Graft versus host disease:**
1. may follow bone marrow transplants
2. may follow blood transfusion
3. occurs in Hodgkin's disease
4. can be suppressed by tetracyclines
5. can be suppressed by cyclophosphamide

6.1   Wound healing is enhanced by the administration of:
1. cortisol
2. zinc
3. aldosterone
4. oxygen
5. vitamin C

PAPER 1

Question number	Answer				
23.1	1. T	2. T	3. T	4. F	5. F
7.24	1. F	2. T	3. F	4. F	5. T
16.1	1. T	2. T	3. T	4. F	5. T
10.3	1. T	2. T	3. F	4. F	5. F
1.3	1. T	2. T	3. T	4. T	5. T
14.14	1. T	2. T	3. F	4. T	5. T
16.4	1. F	2. F	3. F	4. F	5. T
20.8	1. T	2. F	3. T	4. F	5. F
21.1	1. F	2. T	3. F	4. F	5. T
3.5	1. T	2. F	3. T	4. F	5. F
4.7	1. F	2. T	3. F	4. T	5. F
4.5	1. F	2. T	3. T	4. T	5. F
24.7	1. F	2. T	3. F	4. T	5. T
3.11	1. T	2. F	3. T	4. F	5. F
6.2	1. T	2. T	3. T	4. F	5. T
17.18	1. F	2. T	3. T	4. F	5. T
18.7	1. F	2. F	3. T	4. F	5. F
7.16	1. F	2. T	3. F	4. T	5. T
7.33	1. T	2. T	3. F	4. F	5. T
6.1	1. F	2. T	3. F	4. T	5. T

PAPER 2

12.11 The following coagulation factors are generated in the liver:
1. Factor II
2. Factor IV
3. Factor VI
4. Factor IX
5. Factor X

16.5 Infarction may occur as a complication in the following diseases:
1. atherosclerosis
2. Monckeberg's sclerosis
3. benign hypertension
4. sickle-cell anaemia
5. idiopathic thrombocytopenic purpura

10.4 Amyloid is deposited most frequently in:
1. liver
2. brain
3. spleen
4. lungs
5. kidneys

7.14 Immune complex disease is associated with:
1. autoimmunity
2. skin graft rejection
3. Pigeon Fancier's lung
4. meningococcal infection
5. talc granuloma

18.4 Primary thyrotoxicosis is always accompanied by:
1. increased iodine uptake by the gland
2. a raised protein bound iodine
3. exophthalmos
4. hypercalcaemia
5. pernicious anaemia

7.3 Bence–Jones proteins are:
1. the heavy chains of immunoglobulins
2. found in the urine in multiple myeloma
3. associated with a monoclonal gammopathy
4. found in the urine in Waldenström's macroglobulinaemia
5. precipitated by boiling

23.2 The virus associated with HIV is:
1. an obligate intracellular virus
2. a commoner infection in haemophiliacs than in normal individuals
3. transmitted from mother to infant
4. related to the visna virus which infects sheep
5. a single genetic form

12.2   Haemolytic jaundice is associated with:
1. an increase in the concentration of bilirubin diglucuronide in the bile
2. the presence of bilirubin in the urine
3. an increase in the serum alkaline phosphatase
4. a decrease in unconjugated bilirubin in the serum
5. an increase in urobilinogen in the urine

7.1   The following substances normally act as antigens, i.e. stimulate antibody production, when administered to humans:
1. dextrans with a molecular weight below 150 000
2. bovine insulin
3. extracts of Primula
4. human thyroglobulin
5. Rh.D antigen

12.8   Gall stones are associated with the following diseases:
1. viral hepatitis
2. cirrhosis of the liver
3. hereditary spherocytosis
4. obesity
5. raised serum triglycerides

22.4   The following are immunosuppressive drugs:
1. azathioprine
2. indomethacin
3. oxyprenolol
4. cyclophosphamide
5. chlorpropamide

24.2   The 'sick cell syndrome' is associated with:
1. cardiac failure following surgery or trauma
2. failure of the sodium pump
3. a rise in the urinary sodium excretion
4. apathy
5. intracellular oedema

17.14   The following biochemical changes occur in pernicious anaemia:
1. a raised serum vitamin B_{12}
2. a normal serum folate
3. a raised serum bilirubin
4. an increased alkaline phosphatase
5. a decreased plasma copper

5.8 **Antibiotics which inhibit the synthesis of mucopeptide in the wall of a bacterium include:**
1. cycloserine
2. cephalosporins
3. neomycin
4. penicillin and its semisynthetic derivatives
5. erythromycin

23.3 **Acute graft versus host disease following bone marrow transplantation is followed by damage to:**
1. the skin
2. the gut
3. the brain
4. the liver
5. the endocrine glands

6.8 **Woven bone is found:**
1. in bone forming in a model of cartilage
2. in fracture haematomas
3. in bones forming in sheets of differentiating mesenchyme
4. replacing lamellar bone in healing fractures
5. surrounding the ends of ununited fractures

20.7 **The metabolic effects following a severe injury include:**
1. respiratory alkalosis
2. accelerated gluconeogenesis
3. mobilisation of fat stores
4. decreased aldosterone secretion
5. protein anabolism

17.7 **The commonest haemolytic disorder in the world is:**
1. congenital spherocytosis
2. disseminated lupus erythematosus
3. malaria
4. G6PD deficiency
5. sickle cell disease

2.12 **Microorganisms which have undergone phagocytosis are killed by:**
1. lecithinase
2. lysozyme
3. lysosomal enzymes
4. lymphokine
5. hydrogen peroxide

5.1   When using an autoclave to sterilize surgical drapes and instruments it is essential that:
1. the load should be tightly packed
2. the containers in which the loads are packed should be impervious to steam
3. air should be completely removed from the chamber prior to the admission of steam
4. a vacuum must be made at the end of the cycle
5. an adequate indication of autoclave efficiency should be included in the load

PAPER 2

Question number   *Answer*

12.11	1. T	2. F	3. F	4. T	5. T
16.5	1. T	2. F	3. F	4. T	5. F
10.4	1. T	2. T	3. T	4. F	5. T
7.14	1. T	2. F	3. T	4. T	5. F
18.4	1. T	2. T	3. F	4. T	5. F
7.3	1. F	2. T	3. T	4. F	5. F
23.2	1. T	2. F	3. T	4. T	5. F
12.2	1. T	2. F	3. F	4. F	5. T
7.1	1. T	2. T	3. F	4. F	5. T
12.8	1. F	2. F	3. T	4. T	5. T
22.4	1. T	2. F	3. F	4. T	5. F
24.2	1. T	2. T	3. F	4. T	5. T
17.14	1. F	2. T	3. T	4. F	5. F
5.8	1. T	2. T	3. F	4. T	5. F
23.3	1. T	2. T	3. F	4. T	5. F
6.8	1. F	2. T	3. T	4. F	5. F
20.7	1. T	2. T	3. T	4. F	5. F
17.7	1. F	2. F	3. T	4. F	5. F
2.12	1. F	2. T	3. T	4. F	5. T
5.1	1. F	2. F	3. T	4. T	5. T

PAPER 3

23.4   AIDS encephalopathy is:
1. an infrequent feature of the disease
2. mainly affects the grey matter
3. associated with rarefaction and vacuolation
4. associated with mental retardation in children
5. caused by CD4+ T-cell deficiency

10.5   The following conditions are particularly associated with the deposition of amyloid:
1. gas gangrene
2. leprosy
3. chronic osteomyelitis
4. Type II diabetes
5. pneumococcal pneumonia

7.35   The following infections are common in immunodeficient patients:
1. *Pneumocystis carinii*
2. diphtheria
3. poliomyelitis
4. cytomegalovirus
5. *Candida albicans*

24.4   The compensatory mechanisms available to preserve the organism as a whole in the 'shock state' include:
1. autoregulation
2. a fall in the pO_2 of the blood
3. decreased pulmonary compliance
4. an increased sympathoadrenal discharge
5. haemoconcentration

17.35   Consecutive clot:
1. occurs in arteries distal to a thrombotic obstruction
2. occurs in the collateral branches of an artery following obstruction to the main vessel
3. occurs in veins after the cessation of blood flow
4. extends proximally to the entrance of the next venous tributary
5. is formed of coralline thrombus

24.3   The chief pathological and physiological changes in 'shock lung' include:
1. intra-alveolar oedema and extravasation of erythrocytes into the alveoli
2. increased pulmonary compliance
3. infection
4. alkalosis
5. patchy opacities on the plain X-ray of the chest

17.32   Thrombocytopenia:
1. may occur as an autoimmune phenomenon
2. is caused by sulphonamides
3. is associated with an increased bleeding time
4. is associated with an increased clotting time
5. the thromboplastin generation test is useful in its recognition

7.29   The following microorganisms are obligate or facultative intracellular parasites:
1. *Mycobacterium tuberculosis*
2. *Clostridium welchii*
3. *Corynebacterium diphtheria*
4. *Leishmania tropica*
5. herpes simplex

16.11   Acute heart failure occurs:
1. in rheumatic fever
2. in rheumatoid arthritis
3. in myxoedema
4. following myocardial infarction
5. in acute nephritis

2.9   The following are the chemical mediators involved in acute inflammation:
1. complement
2. histamine
3. insulin
4. bradykinin
5. lymphokine

22.7   The following immunosuppressive agents are purine or pyrimidine analogues:
1. cyclosporine
2. azathioprine
3. methotrexate
4. actinomycin
5. prednisone

7.10   Antibodies may be detected in vitro by:
1. precipitation
2. complement fixation
3. lymphokine production
4. lymphocyte transformation test
5. RIA, ELISA and RAST

24.10   Serum levels of HBsAg may be high in:
1. lepromatous leprosy
2. tuberculosis
3. Down's syndrome
4. heroin addicts
5. malignant melanoma

3.2   The following belong to the mononuclear phagocyte system:
1. macrophages
2. mast cells
3. epithelioid cells
4. fibroblasts
5. Küpffer cells

7.26   The following are the chief characteristics of delayed hypersensitivity reactions:
1. the development of a polymorphonuclear leucocyte infiltrate
2. the reaction has reached its maximum intensity at 4 hours
3. an individual can be passively sensitised with serum
4. it is associated with T-lymphocyte function
5. complement activation is an essential factor

7.22   The following are, or contain, autoantibodies:
1. cryoglobulins
2. rheumatoid factor
3. migration inhibitory factor
4. antinuclear factor
5. transfer factor

20.10   Severe pyloric stenosis is accompanied by the following biochemical changes:
1. a fall in the effective blood volume
2. a fall in the concentration of plasma sodium
3. a rise in pCO_2
4. hypotonic urine
5. hyperkalaemia

17.25   The plasma prothrombin time is increased in:
1. hepatocellular disease
2. obstructive jaundice
3. haemophilia
4. Christmas disease
5. following splenectomy

10.6   Secondary amyloidosis occurs in the following conditions:
1. familial Mediterranean fever
2. thalassaemia
3. sickle-cell disease
4. multiple myeloma
5. rheumatoid arthritis

14.10   The commonest tumours of the central nervous system arise from:
1. the meninges
2. primary tumours elsewhere in the body
3. neuroglia
4. the blood vessels
5. nerve cells

PAPER 3

Question number	Answer				
23.4	1. F	2. F	3. T	4. T	5. F
10.5	1. F	2. T	3. T	4. T	5. F
7.35	1. T	2. F	3. F	4. T	5. T
24.4	1. T	2. F	3. F	4. T	5. F
17.35	1. F	2. F	3. T	4. T	5. F
24.3	1. T	2. F	3. T	4. F	5. T
17.32	1. T	2. T	3. T	4. F	5. F
7.29	1. T	2. F	3. F	4. T	5. T
16.11	1. T	2. F	3. F	4. T	5. T
2.9	1. T	2. T	3. F	4. T	5. F
22.7	1. F	2. T	3. F	4. F	5. F
7.10	1 T	2. T	3. F	4. F	5. T
24.10	1. T	2. F	3. T	4. T	5. F
3.2	1. T	2. F	3. T	4. F	5. T
7.26	1. F	2. F	3. F	4. T	5. F
7.22	1. T	2. T	3. F	4. T	5. F
20.10	1. T	2. F	3. T	4. F	5. F
17.25	1. T	2. T	3. F	4. F	5. F
10.6	1. T	2. F	3. F	4. T	5. T
14.10	1. F	2. T	3. T	4. F	5. F

PAPER 4

11.5   Haemosiderosis differs from haemochromatosis in that:
1. the former is more common in the Bantu
2. the latter is due to the excessive absorption of iron and the former to excessive intake
3. in the former the excessive iron is mainly deposited in the parenchymal cells, whereas in the latter the excess iron is deposited chiefly in the macrophages of the liver, spleen and bone marrow
4. in the former cirrhosis does not develop
5. in the latter the level of plasma transferrin is abnormally high

3.9   Epithelioid cell granuloma formation is associated with the following diseases:
1. ulcerative colitis
2. Crohn's disease
3. chronic glomerulo-nephritis
4. toxoplasmosis
5. sarcoidosis

9.7   Osteoporosis differs from osteomalacia in that:
1. the radiographic density of the skeleton is reduced in the former and not the latter
2. the remaining bone in the former presents a normal histological appearance
3. major changes occur in the epiphyses in the former
4. pseudofractures are commoner in the former than the latter
5. excess osteoid tissue is present in the former

19.7   Uretero-colic anastomosis is followed by:
1. ascending pyelonephritis
2. absorption of ammonium salts
3. absorption of urea from the colon
4. metabolic alkalosis
5. hyperkalaemia

7.11   Hypogammaglobulinaemia may occur in the following conditions:
1. prematurity and infancy
2. gluten sensitive enteropathy
3. Di George syndrome
4. autoimmune thyroiditis
5. Hodgkin's lymphomas

20.2 The percentage of total body water in any individual is influenced by:
1. the lean body mass
2. the activity of the adrenal cortex
3. the sodium content of the diet
4. thyroid activity
5. vomiting

3.1 Necrosis occurs as a concomitant feature of chronic inflammation in:
1. leprosy
2. tuberculosis
3. syphilis
4. actinomycosis
5. coccidiomycosis

7.8 The germinal centres of lymph nodes:
1. participate in cell-mediated immunity
2. contain macrophages and plasma cells
3. after producing B cells discharge these via the subcapsular (marginal) sinus into the general circulation
4. enlarge in chronic infectious diseases
5. are absent in humans suffering from congenital thymic aplasia

23.5 Immunosuppression can be achieved by:
1. cyclosporine
2. rapamycin
3. monoclonal antibodies
4. poor renal function
5. blood transfusion prior to surgery

7.19 Serum sickness:
1. can be caused by an injection of diphtheria antitoxin
2. is common following immunization against tetanus
3. can follow an injection of penicillin
4. is mediated by immune complexes
5. may involve IgE

6.5 Post operative infection delays wound healing because:
1. the wound becomes packed with leucocytes
2. many of the organisms involved produce spreading factors which may destroy the intercellular ground substance
3. collagen is destroyed
4. capillary loops fail to develop
5. fibroblasts are diminished in number

17.12 The following abnormalities occur in pernicious anaemia:
1. a low haemoglobin
2. a decreased mean corpuscular haemoglobin (MCH)
3. an increased reticulocyte count
4. antibodies to the parietal cells of the stomach
5. a decrease in the circulating level of vitamin B$_{12}$

17.13 In pernicious anaemia the following pathological changes may be seen:
1. haemosiderosis
2. atrophy of the gastric mucosa
3. a decrease in the volume of red marrow in the long bones
4. extramedullary haemopoiesis
5. demyelination of the lateral and dorsal columns, not associated with gliosis

3.10 Organised epithelioid cell granulomas develop in the following infections:
1. leprosy
2. syphilis
3. ankylostomiasis
4. ascariasis
5. schistosomiasis

23.6 Kaposi's sarcoma is:
1. not as common as non-Hodgkin's lymphoma in patients suffering from AIDS
2. different in the sporadic form from that occurring in AIDS
3. histologically identical in both the sporadic and AIDS-related forms
4. not associated with transplantation
5. related to haemangiosarcoma

12.1 Obstruction of the common bile duct is associated with the following biochemical abnormalities:
1. a greater increase in the serum concentration of bilirubin diglucuronide than bilirubin monoglucuronide
2. a decrease in the serum concentration of unconjugated bilirubin
3. a decrease in the faecal stercobilinogen content
4. an increase in faecal fat
5. an increase in urinary urobilinogen

17.28   Haemorrhagic lesions may occur as a result of:
1. vitamin B deficiency
2. vitamin C deficiency
3. retinol deficiency
4. the nephrotic syndrome
5. penicillin therapy

15.7   The following infections may be successfully prevented by the administration of a vaccine:
1. herpes simplex
2. rabies
3. Lassa fever
4. poliomyelitis
5. yellow fever

22.8   Chlorambucil, a potent cytotoxic agent, causes:
1. bone marrow depression
2. indirect interference with mitosis
3. inhibition of purine synthesis
4. binding of DNA strands
5. inhibition of protein synthesis

18.8   The Zollinger–Ellison syndrome is associated with:
1. β-cell tumours of the pancreas
2. chronic duodenal ulceration
3. cholereiform diarrhoea
4. parathyroid adenomata
5. phaeochromocytoma

PAPER 4

Question number   *Answer*

Question number	Answer				
11.5	1. F	2. T	3. F	4. T	5. F
3.9	1. F	2. T	3. F	4. T	5. T
9.7	1. F	2. T	3. F	4. F	5. F
19.7	1. T	2. T	3. T	4. F	5. F
7.11	1. T	2. T	3. F	4. F	5. T
20.2	1. T	2. T	3. F	4. T	5. T
3.1	1. F	2. T	3. T	4. T	5. T
7.8	1. F	2. T	3. F	4. T	5. F
23.5	1. T	2. T	3. T	4. T	5. T
7.19	1. T	2. F	3. T	4. T	5. T
6.5	1. F	2. F	3. T	4. F	5. F
17.12	1. T	2. F	3. F	4. T	5. T
17.13	1. T	2. T	3. F	4. T	5. T
3.10	1. T	2. T	3. F	4. F	5. T
23.6	1. F	2. T	3. T	4. F	5. F
12.1	1. F	2. F	3. T	4. T	5. F
17.28	1. F	2. T	3. F	4. F	5. T
15.7	1. F	2. T	3. F	4. T	5. T
22.8	1. T	2. T	3. F	4. T	5. T
18.8	1. T	2. T	3. T	4. T	5. F

PAPER 5

7.18   The production of antibody is essential to host resistance in the following infections:
1. leprosy
2. *Streptococcus pneumoniae*
3. variola
4. tetanus
5. malaria

13.10   The following are specific markers for certain specific types of malignancy:
1. 5-HIAA
2. α-fetoprotein
3. Bence–Jones protein
4. chorionic gonadotrophin
5. carcinoembryonic antigen

2.14   Septicaemia is associated with:
1. a bacteraemia
2. toxaemia
3. the multiplication of bacteria in the blood stream
4. invasion of the blood stream by organisms multiplying elsewhere, e.g. the peritoneum
5. multiple haemorrhagic foci in the tissues

2.10   The following substances are involved in acute inflammation:
1. peptides
2. lectins
3. plasmin
4. LATS
5. PGE_1

17.20   Chronic lymphocytic leukaemia is associated with:
1. a marked increase in the number of lymphocytes in the peripheral blood
2. is not associated with hepatosplenomegaly
3. in some cases thrombocytopenia
4. an increase in the serum globulin concentration
5. chromosomal abnormalities

4.2   General factors predisposing to wound infection include:
1. uncontrolled diabetes
2. hypogammaglobulinaemia
3. low platelet count
4. agranulocytopenia
5. eosinophilia

2.11   Phagocytosis is promoted by:
1. hyaluronidase
2. neuraminidase
3. the hexose monophosphate shunt
4. immunoglobulin
5. complement

23.7   The following grafts are rejected:
1. autografts
2. isografts
3. allografts
4. xenografts
5. corneal grafts

2.8   The main components of the pyogenic membrane are:
1. eosinophils
2. capillary loops
3. hyaluronidase
4. polymorphonuclear leucocytes
5. fibroblasts

6.7   Wound healing may be governed by the following:
1. trephones
2. vitamin D
3. chalones
4. mineralocorticoids
5. the availability of sulphur containing aminoacids

19.2   The renal control of acid base balance is a function of the:
1. loop of Henlé
2. proximal tubule
3. glomerulus
4. distal tubule
5. collecting tubule

2.1   Acute inflammation can be caused by:
1. *Streptococcus pneumoniae*
2. *Mycobacterium tuberculosis*
3. *Neisseria meningitidis*
4. *Mycobacterium leprae*
5. *Borrelia vincenti*

7.17   Complement activation takes place:
1. in the presence of endotoxin
2. as part of the tuberculin reaction
3. by more than one pathway
4. in anaphylaxis
5. by antigen IgA interaction

12.4 In liver failure the following biochemical abnormalities may be found:
1. a decrease in the plasma albumin concentration
2. an increase in the plasma globulin
3. an increase in the blood ammonium concentration
4. a rise in the blood urea
5. impaired glucose tolerance

5.4 Chemical agents used as disinfectants and antiseptics include the following compounds:
1. the phenols
2. isopropyl alcohol
3. the halogens
4. the soaps
5. derivatives of salicylic acid

7.34 The following can cause immunological unresponsiveness:
1. immunological tolerance
2. immunological enhancement
3. Freund's adjuvant
4. T lymphocytes
5. antigen-antibody complexes

14.3 Neoplastic disease may be associated with the following conditions:
1. dermatomyositis
2. acanthosis nigricans
3. necrobiosis lipoidica
4. thrombophlebitis migrans
5. polyarteritis nodosa

23.8 HIV infection is associated with:
1. a reduction in the number of B cells
2. hypergammaglobulinaemia
3. increased tuberculin skin test reactivity
4. cytokine abnormalities
5. autoimmunity

6.9 The healing of a closed fracture may be associated with the following pathological consequences:
1. myositis ossificans
2. pseudoarthrosis
3. osteomyelitis
4. osteosarcoma
5. renal calculi

16.3   The following conditions are associated with hyperlipidaemia:
1. familial hypercholesteraemia
2. the nephrotic syndrome
3. Von Gierke's syndrome
4. hyperaldosteronism
5. thyrotoxicosis

PAPER 5

Question number	Answer				
7.18	1. F	2. T	3. T	4. T	5. F
13.10	1. T	2. F	3. T	4. T	5. F
2.14	1. F	2. T	3. T	4. T	5. T
2.10	1. T	2. T	3. T	4. F	5. T
17.20	1. T	2. F	3. T	4. F	5. T
4.2	1. T	2. T	3. T	4. T	5. F
2.11	1. F	2. F	3. F	4. T	5. T
23.7	1. F	2. F	3. T	4. T	5. F
2.8	1. F	2. T	3. F	4. T	5. T
6.7	1. T	2. F	3. T	4. F	5. T
19.2	1. F	2. F	3. F	4. T	5. F
2.1	1. T	2. T	3. T	4. F	5. T
7.17	1. T	2. F	3. T	4. F	5. F
12.4	1. T	2. T	3. T	4. F	5. T
5.4	1. T	2. T	3. T	4. T	5. F
7.34	1. T	2. T	3. F	4. T	5. T
14.3	1. T	2. T	3. F	4. T	5. F
23.8	1. F	2. T	3. F	4. T	5. F
6.9	1. T	2. T	3. F	4. F	5. T
16.3	1. T	2. T	3. T	4. F	5. F

PAPER 6

7.9   Lymphokines, soluble factors released from primed lymphocytes in contact with an antigen are important in:
1. anaphylaxis
2. immune complex disease
3. macrophage activation
4. graft rejection
5. the involvement of the activation of natural killer cells

12.9   Severe liver failure is associated with:
1. mucosal bleeding
2. encephalopathy
3. bronchopneumonia
4. venous thrombosis
5. decreased resistance to infection

23.9   Chronic renal allograft rejection is a process:
1. affecting about 10–30% of long-surviving grafts
2. characterized by proliferative stenosis of the arteries
3. in which cellular infiltrates and fibrinoid necrosis occurs
4. which can be reversed by medical treatment
5. which requires graft replacement

15.6   The Hepatitis B virus:
1. is transmitted by the oral route
2. is transmitted by dogs
3. is common in renal dialysis units
4. is the cause of Burkitt's lymphoma
5. causes immune complex disease

21.7   The Coombs test is used for detecting:
1. rheumatoid factor
2. antinuclear factor
3. haemolytic autoantibodies
4. cold agglutinins
5. rhesus antibodies

15.2   Encephalitis may be a complication of the following virus infections:
1. Epstein–Barr virus
2. measles virus
3. rubella virus
4. herpes virus
5. adenovirus

17.29 Disseminated intravascular coagulation occurs as a complication of:
1. many obstetrical complications
2. malignant disease
3. polycythaemia vera
4. the overadministration of thrombokinase
5. endotoxaemic shock

9.3 The destruction of bone is associated with the following biochemical changes:
1. an increased secretion of hydroxyproline in the urine
2. an elevated alkaline phosphatase
3. an elevated acid phosphatase
4. an elevated serum calcium
5. depression of the serum phosphate

7.7 Autoimmunity:
1. occurs because of a breakdown in the ability of the body to distinguish between self and non-self
2. is a rare cause of infertility in the male
3. is not involved in the development of pernicious anaemia
4. is important in the pathogenesis of lupus erythematosus
5. does not result in immune complex disease

14.7 The findings of the following substances in excessive quantities in the blood may be due to the presence of a specific type of tumour:
1. noradrenaline
2. 5-hydroxytryptamine
3. carcinoembryonic antigen
4. prostaglandins
5. calcium

17.19 Chronic myeloid leukaemia differs from chronic lymphatic leukaemia in that:
1. in the former the predominant white cell in the circulation is the leucocyte
2. the total white count is higher in chronic lymphatic leukaemia
3. in the former the proliferating marrow cells possess the Philadelphia chromosome
4. the latter is more common in an older age group than is the former
5. the former disease tends to develop into a more aggressive type of acute leukaemia

2.7   **The magnitude of leucocyte migration into an area infected with bacteria is governed by:**
1. the type of organism causing the inflammatory lesion
2. chemotaxins
3. the C5a complement component
4. the phosphatase levels in the inflamed area
5. the formation of pus

10.8   **Amyloidosis may be associated with elevated levels of the following serum proteins:**
1. β-lipoprotein
2. SAA
3. IgD
4. M-protein
5. β-microglobulin

18.5   **Abnormal aggregation of lymphocytes occurs in the thyroid in the following pathological conditions:**
1. follicular carcinoma
2. medullary carcinoma
3. lymphadenoid goitre
4. Heidel's struma
5. primary thyrotoxicosis

24.9   **Chromosome abnormalities may occur:**
1. in Klinefelter's syndrome
2. following treatment with methotrexate
3. as a result of ionising radiation
4. in Down's syndrome
5. in Christmas disease

23.10   **Hyperacute rejection is:**
1. a condition associated with a T-cell mediated reaction
2. a condition recognised at operation
3. associated with the Schwartzmann reaction
4. a condition mediated by preformed antibodies
5. a condition seen in multiparous women

7.27 Maximum changes occur in the following skin reactions within 24 to 48 hours:
1. Schwartzmann reaction
2. Arthus reaction
3. tuberculin reaction
4. contact patch test
5. skin allograft rejection

14.6 Exfoliative cytology is useful for the diagnosis of:
1. meningioma
2. bronchial cancer
3. multiple myeloma
4. cervical cancer
5. vesical cancer

24.1 The following are referred to as 'Incomplete Antibodies':
1. IgG anti-D
2. IgM anti-D
3. anti-A isohaemagglutinin
4. the Wassermann antibody
5. tetanus antitoxin

14.5 The following tumours may secrete hormones:
1. carcinoid tumours
2. choriocarcinoma
3. benign teratoma of the ovary
4. monodermal teratoma of the ovary
5. seminoma

PAPER 6

Question number   *Answer*

7.9	1. F	2. F	3. T	4. T	5. T
12.9	1. T	2. T	3. T	4. F	5. T
23.9	1. T	2. T	3. F	4. F	5. T
15.6	1. T	2. F	3. T	4. F	5. T
21.7	1. F	2. F	3. T	4. T	5. T
15.2	1. T	2. T	3. T	4. T	5. F
17.29	1. T	2. T	3. F	4. F	5. T
9.3	1. T	2. T	3. F	4. T	5. T
7.7	1. T	2. T	3. F	4. T	5. T
14.7	1. T	2. T	3. T	4. F	5. T
17.19	1. T	2. F	3. T	4. F	5. T
2.7	1. T	2. T	3. T	4. F	5. T
10.8	1. F	2. T	3. F	4. T	5. F
18.5	1. F	2. F	3. T	4. F	5. T
24.9	1. T	2. F	3. T	4. T	5. F
23.10	1. F	2. T	3. F	4. T	5. T
7.27	1. F	2. F	3. T	4. T	5. F
14.6	1. F	2. T	3. F	4. T	5. T
24.1	1. T	2. F	3. F	4. F	5. F
14.5	1. T	2. T	3. F	4. T	5. T

PAPER 7

23.11 Which of the following statements regarding HIV infection is true:
1. infection with HIV is followed by a short incubation period and by a rapidly progressive illness ending in a fatal outcome
2. it is associated with the formation of giant cells
3. the virus expresses specific trophism for the haemopoetic and nervous systems
4. the risk of infection by blood transfusion has been completely eliminated
5. the virus is surrounded by a lipid membrane

2.13 Pus contains:
1. lipids
2. fibrin
3. collagen
4. plasma cells
5. polymorphonuclear leucocytes

5.3 Differences between disinfectants and antiseptics are as follows:
1. the latter are more harmful to living tissue cells
2. antiseptics free inanimate objects from vegetative organisms whereas disinfectants are used for the local removal of pathogenic bacteria from the tissues
3. the former are more readily inactivated by contact with proteinaceous material such as blood
4. the speed of action of disinfectants can be accelerated by raising the temperature whereas the action of antiseptics can only be intensified by increasing their concentration
5. there are specific differences in the mode of action of both groups of compounds

4.8 The major pathogens in postoperative chest infections are:
1. *Haemophilus influenzae*
2. *Streptococcus pyogenes*
3. *Mycobacterium tuberculosis*
4. *Staphylococcus aureus*
5. *Streptococcus pneumoniae*

22.5 The following compounds may be used as anti–cancer agents:
1. azathioprine
2. methotrexate
3. actinomycin D
4. chlorambucil
5. cyclosporin A

21.4 An immediate reaction to a blood transfusion may be caused by the following:
1. hypercalcaemia
2. air embolus
3. bacterial endotoxins
4. anaphylaxis
5. hypokalaemia

14.12 The interphase is:
1. situated between the prophase and metaphase
2. a resting stage between cell division
3. associated with growth of a cell
4. accompanied by the accumulation of RNA
5. situated between the anaphase and the telophase

3.7 The following predispose to the development of tuberculosis:
1. HLA–B27
2. sarcoidosis
3. silicosis
4. avitaminosis D
5. malnutrition

16.10 The following congenital anomalies of the heart are accompanied by continuous cyanosis:
1. complete transposition of the great vessels
2. uncomplicated patent ductus arteriosus
3. coarctation of the aorta
4. double aortic arch
5. tetralogy of Fallot

19.4 The nephrotic syndrome is accompanied by:
1. decreased glomerular capillary permeability
2. oedema
3. a loss of 10 g or more of plasma protein daily
4. hypolipidaemia
5. abundant cortical deposits of neutral fat and anisotropic lipids

3.6 Giant cells are characteristically found in the pathological lesions associated with the following diseases:
1. actinomycosis
2. schistosomiasis
3. primary biliary cirrhosis
4. lepromatous leprosy
5. Hodgkin's disease

23.12 The major histocompatibility complex (MHC) in man:
1. is situated on chromosome 6
2. the genes are grouped into three types
3. is involved in antigen presentation
4. shows a positive association with Hodgkin's disease, multiple sclerosis and ankylosing spondylitis
5. is tested for by the laboratory on a serum sample

2.2 The following agents produce an acute inflammatory reaction in unsensitised individuals:
1. lipopolysaccharide
2. albumin
3. ultra-violet light
4. insulin
5. carbon particles

9.4 Hypercalcaemia and hypercalciuria is caused by:
1. osteolytic secondary deposits in bone
2. hypervitaminosis D, often referred to as vitamin D intoxication
3. parathyroid tumours
4. tumours of adrenal medulla
5. primary carcinoma of the kidney restricted to the kidney

16.2 Cholesterol is believed to be of great importance in the development of atherosclerosis because:
1. low plasma cholesterol concentrations are associated with relative freedom from atherosclerotic heart disease
2. high concentrations of cholesterol occur in the atherosclerotic plaques
3. patients suffering from steatorrhoea develop atherosclerosis at a younger age than normal individuals
4. diabetes is associated with an increased incidence of atherosclerosis
5. atherosclerosis can be induced in non-human primates by dietary measures which increase the concentration of cholesterol in the plasma

5.9 Ototoxicity is a well recognised complication following the administration of:
1. streptomycin
2. gentamicin
3. neomycin
4. bacitracin
5. erythromycin

13.7   The following infections are associated with the development of cancer:
1. clostridial infections
2. HBV infection
3. EBV infection
4. chlamydial infections
5. schistosomiasis

22.2   The effect(s) of ionising irradiation:
1. are increased by sulphydryl reagents
2. are increased by increased oxygen tension
3. is mainly upon mitochondria
4. is to cause diarrhoea
5. is to cause a deficiency of clotting factors

17.34   Thrombocytopenic purpura differs from non-thrombocytopenic purpura in that:
1. in the former condition the platelet count is reduced
2. in the latter the main defect is in the capillaries
3. the former may follow systemic disease
4. the latter may result from allergy
5. petechiae occur in the former but not in the latter

7.15   The third component of complement is:
1. a factor in phagocytosis
2. an anaphylatoxin
3. chemotactic
4. a migration inhibition factor
5. an interferon

PAPER 7

Question number	Answer				
23.11	1. F	2. T	3. T	4. F	5. T
2.13	1. T	2. T	3. F	4. F	5. T
5.3	1. F	2. F	3. F	4. F	5. F
4.8	1. T	2. F	3. F	4. T	5. T
22.5	1. F	2. T	3. T	4. T	5. F
21.4	1. F	2. T	3. T	4. T	5. F
14.12	1. F	2. T	3. T	4. T	5. F
3.7	1. F	2. F	3. T	4. F	5. T
16.10	1. T	2. F	3. F	4. F	5. T
19.4	1. F	2. T	3. T	4. F	5. T
3.6	1. F	2. F	3. T	4. F	5. T
23.12	1. T	2. T	3. T	4. T	5. F
2.2	1. T	2. F	3. T	4. F	5. F
9.4	1. T	2. T	3. T	4. F	5. F
16.2	1. T	2. T	3. F	4. F	5. T
5.9	1. T	2. T	3. T	4. F	5. F
13.7	1. F	2. T	3. T	4. F	5. T
22.2	1. F	2. T	3. F	4. T	5. F
17.34	1. T	2. T	3. T	4. T	5. F
7.15	1. T	2. T	3. T	4. F	5. F

PAPER 8

20.1   The major differences between the plasma and the interstitial fluid are in:
1. the concentration of sodium
2. the concentration of calcium
3. the bicarbonate concentration
4. the protein content
5. the organic acid concentration

13.1   A hereditary predisposition to the development of tumours occurs in the following sites:
1. retina
2. colon
3. uterus
4. skin
5. stomach

14.1   A tumour may be defined as:
1. an abnormal mass of tissue
2. a growth of tissue which exceeds and is uncoordinated with that of normal tissues
3. a growth of tissue which is limited and coordinated with that of the rest of the body
4. an abnormal increase in the cells of a tissue
5. a malformation in which the various tissues of the part are present in improper proportions or distribution

15.3   Inclusion bodies are found in the following viral infections:
1. measles
2. yellow fever
3. rabies
4. hepatitis B
5. smallpox

17.10   Polycythaemia occurs in:
1. congenital cyanotic heart disease
2. tumours of the renal parenchyma, renal carcinoma
3. the carcinoid syndrome
4. lead poisoning
5. hypoxia

23.13   Infection with HIV can cause:
1. an illness resembling acute glandular fever
2. persistent generalized lymphadenopathy
3. neurological complications
4. monoclonal B-cell activation
5. antibody formation within 7 days of exposure to infection

14.13 The embryonic tumours of infancy include:
1. nephroblastoma
2. osteogenic sarcoma (osteosarcoma)
3. medulloblastoma
4. cholangiocarcinoma
5. lympho-epithelioma

24.5 Which among the following are protozoal infections:
1. hydatid disease
2. trypanosomiasis
3. giardiasis
4. schistosomiasis
5. filariasis

3.4 Accumulation of macrophages is a prominent histological feature of the lesions produced by the following diseases:
1. leishmaniasis
2. extrinsic allergic alveolitis
3. Gaucher's disease
4. legionnaire's disease
5. Letterer–Siwe's disease

10.9 Amyloid reacts with the following stains:
1. thioflavine-T
2. fluoroscein isothiocyanate
3. methyl violet
4. methyl green
5. Congo red

17.22 An enlarged lymph node which is excised is found by histological examination to be packed with tubercles consisting of epithelioid cells and giant cells. The tuberculin and Heaf test are negative. Which of the following diseases should then be considered as the probable cause of the lymphadenopathy:
1. Hodgkin's disease
2. tuberculosis
3. sarcoidosis
4. syphilis
5. toxoplasmosis

9.8 Urinary hydroxyproline excretion may be increased in:
1. Paget's disease of bone
2. Cushing's syndrome
3. hypopituitarism in children
4. hyperthyroidism
5. extensive fractures

17.11   Megaloblastic anaemia may be caused by:
1. atrophy or ablation of the gastric mucosa
2. infestation with *Diphyllobothrium latum*
3. lesions involving the terminal ileum
4. over–enthusiastic use of purgatives
5. small bowel blind loops

5.7   Bacteria resistant to benzyl penicillin include:
1. penicillinase-producing organisms
2. the majority of Gram-negative bacteria
3. Gram-positive anaerobic spore forming organisms
4. the Bacteroides
5. *Streptococcus pneumoniae*

20.6   Pure water depletion in the surgical patient follows:
1. persistent vomiting
2. dysphagia
3. severe diarrhoea
4. persistent fever
5. the development of diabetes insipidus

9.6   The sites in which metastatic calcification occurs are:
1. the kidney
2. the wall of the inferior vena cava
3. old tuberculous lesions
4. atheroma
5. the cornea

7.31   The following cells play an important role in skin allograft rejection:
1. polymorphonuclear leucocytes
2. macrophages
3. mast cells
4. B lymphocytes
5. T lymphocytes

2.6   The following cell types are involved in acute inflammation:
1. polymorphonuclear leucocytes
2. lymphocytes
3. endothelial cells
4. epithelioid cells
5. mast cells

1.1   Disuse atrophy follows:
1. blockage of the duct of an exocrine gland
2. immobilisation of a joint
3. interference with the nerve supply to the muscles controlling joint movement
4. interference with the blood supply
5. the diminished secretion of trophic hormones

17.2   Alterations in the structure of the Hb molecule give rise to the following diseases:
1. haemolytic disease of the newborn
2. sickle-cell anaemia
3. paroxysmal cold haemoglobinuria
4. paroxysmal nocturnal haemoglobinuria
5. thalassaemia major

PAPER 8

Question number	Answer				
20.1	1. T	2. F	3. F	4. T	5. F
13.1	1. T	2. T	3. F	4. T	5. F
14.1	1. T	2. T	3. F	4. F	5. F
15.3	1. T	2. T	3. T	4. F	5. T
17.10	1. T	2. T	3. F	4. F	5. T
23.13	1. T	2. T	3. T	4. F	5. F
14.13	1. T	2. F	3. T	4. F	5. F
24.5	1. F	2. T	3. T	4. F	5. F
3.4	1. T	2. F	3. T	4. F	5. T
10.9	1. T	2. F	3. T	4. F	5. T
17.22	1. F	2. F	3. T	4. F	5. F
9.8	1. T	2. F	3. F	4. T	5. T
17.11	1. T	2. T	3. T	4. F	5. T
5.7	1. T	2. T	3. F	4. T	5. F
20.6	1. F	2. T	3. F	4. T	5. T
9.6	1. T	2. F	3. F	4. F	5. T
7.31	1. F	2. T	3. F	4. F	5. T
2.6	1. T	2. F	3. T	4. F	5. T
1.1	1. T	2. T	3. F	4. F	5. F
17.2	1. F	2. T	3. F	4. F	5. T

PAPER 9

7.6   Macrophages:
1. are not involved in the recognition of antigens
2. do not secrete lysosomal enzymes
3. carry receptors on their surface
4. are involved in the tuberculin reaction
5. play an important role in graft rejection

11.2   Patchy skin pigmentation occurs in the following conditions:
1. Peutz–Jeghers syndrome
2. familial polyposis
3. Addison's disease
4. purpura
5. vitiligo

9.9   The following conditions may be described as metabolic bone disease:
1. osteoporosis
2. Paget's disease
3. osteomalacia
4. osteopetrosis
5. ostoitis fibrosa cystica

24.6   Mosquitoes transmit the following diseases:
1. schistosomiasis
2. leishmaniasis
3. dengue
4. yellow fever
5. malaria

18.10   Diabetes insipidus is associated with:
1. the oversecretion of vasopressin
2. polydipsia
3. a urine specific gravity greater than 1020
4. head injury
5. metastatic cancer

4.9   The following bacteria are commonly found in infected wounds following colonic operations:
1. *Escherichia coli*
2. *Neisseriae meningitidis*
3. *Streptococcus pyogenes*
4. *Streptococcus faecalis*
5. *Bacteroides fragilis*

20.3   **The renin–angiotensin–aldosterone system regulates:**
1. potassium balance
2. sodium balance
3. fluid volume
4. blood pressure
5. nitrogen balance

9.1   **The normal level of ionised calcium in the plasma is maintained by the following mechanisms:**
1. the secretion of calcitonin
2. the presence of 1,25 $(OH)_2 D_3$
3. parathyroid hormone secretion
4. renal tubular conservation
5. the circulating level of magnesium

7.13   **The Arthus reaction:**
1. is associated with marked migration of polymorphonuclear leucocytes into the affected tissues
2. the relative concentration of antigen-antibody is of no importance in this reaction
3. is a delayed hypersensitivity reaction
4. is associated with vascular damage
5. is similar to the Schwartzmann reaction

11.1   **Generalized pigmentation of the skin occurs in:**
1. carcinoma of the head of the pancreas
2. idiopathic hereditary haemochromatosis
3. argyria
4. arsenic poisoning
5. black liver disease

14.9   **Hormone dependency may be exhibited by the following tumours:**
1. malignant melanoma
2. prostatic carcinoma
3. follicular carcinoma of the thyroid
4. bronchial carcinoma
5. retinoblastoma

23.14   **The so-called 'Second Set' phenomenon:**
1. occurs in an animal or human who has not previously rejected an allograft
2. occurs after a latent period of several days
3. depends on the graft antigenicity being recognised by the host T cells
4. can be demonstrated in both man and animals
5. can be delayed by prior irradiation of the graft

22.6   The following compounds are alkylating agents:
1. azathioprine
2. methotrexate
3. cyclophosphamide
4. phenylalanine mustard
5. tetracycline

7.4   T lymphocytes:
1. are immunoglobulin-secreting cells
2. are found in the paracortical area of lymph nodes
3. are involved in contact dermatitis
4. are not involved in protection against tuberculosis
5. secrete lymphokines

15.4   The following are DNA containing viruses:
1. rhinovirus
2. herpes virus
3. vaccinia
4. yellow fever
5. influenza

13.6   The following occupations have been, or remain associated with, a high risk of cancer:
1. coal mining
2. nickel workers
3. asbestos workers
4. beryllium workers
5. tobacco industry

20.9   Hypocalcaemia occurs:
1. following surgical damage or removal of the parathyroid glands
2. following fractures of the long bones
3. during attacks of acute pancreatitis
4. following head injury
5. in association with hypomagnesaemia

7.2   The following statements are true or false:
1. IgA is produced at mucous surfaces
2. IgM has a molecular weight 150 000
3. IgE is the anaphylactic antibody
4. antibody specificity depends on the constant regions of the F(ab) fragment
5. immunoglobulin synthesis is dependent on thymic integrity in neonatal life

7.38   Haptoglobins:
1. bind to the body's own proteins to make them immunogenic
2. are immunoglobulins
3. bind to free haemoglobin
4. are controlled by genetic factors
5. can bind rheumatoid factor

13.5 **The following chemicals are carcinogens, i.e. require metabolic conversion to become carcinogenic:**
1. 1.2.5.6 dibenzanthrazine
2. cyclophosphamide
3. β-naphthylamine
4. acetyl salicyclic acid
5. 4-dimethylamino-azobenzene

PAPER 9

Question number	Answer				
7.6	1. F	2. F	3. T	4. T	5. F
11.2	1. T	2. F	3. F	4. T	5. F
9.9	1. T	2. F	3. T	4. T	5. T
24.6	1. F	2. F	3. T	4. T	5. T
18.10	1. F	2. T	3. F	4. T	5. T
4.9	1. T	2. F	3. T	4. T	5. T
20.3	1. T	2. T	3. T	4. T	5. F
9.1	1. T	2. T	3. T	4. T	5. F
7.13	1. T	2. F	3. F	4. T	5. F
11.1	1. T	2. T	3. T	4. F	5. F
14.9	1. T	2. T	3. T	4. F	5. F
23.14	1. F	2. F	3. T	4. T	5. T
22.6	1. F	2. F	3. T	4. T	5. F
7.4	1. F	2. T	3. T	4. F	5. T
15.4	1. F	2. T	3. T	4. F	5. F
13.6	1. F	2. T	3. T	4. F	5. F
20.9	1. T	2. F	3. T	4. F	5. T
7.2	1. T	2. F	3. T	4. F	5. F
7.38	1. T	2. F	3. T	4. T	5. F
13.5	1. F	2. F	3. T	4. F	5. T

PAPER 10

23.15 Rejection of liver transplants is associated with:
1. arterial lesions
2. cholestasis
3. opportunistic infection
4. autoimmune chronic active hepatitis
5. multiple sclerosis

7.5 The major histocompatibility complex (MHC) in man:
1. is situated on chromosome 6
2. has three loci controlling five groups of histocompatibility antigens
3. is involved in the expression of immune response (Ir) genes
4. shows a positive association with Hodgkin's disease, multiple sclerosis and ankylosing spondylitis
5. is tested for by the laboratory on a serum sample

7.37 A non-specific depression of the tuberculin reaction occurs in:
1. influenza
2. measles
3. sarcoidosis
4. leprosy
5. ulcerative colitis

13.2 Recognised precancerous conditions include:
1. the intestinal polyps of the small bowel present in the Peutz–Jeghers syndrome
2. the colonic polyps of familial polyposis
3. xeroderma pigmentosum
4. Bowen's disease
5. molluscum sebaceum

12.6 Excessive cholesterol is excreted by the hepatocytes:
1. when the diet contains excessive amounts of polyunsaturated fatty acids
2. in response to excessive secretion of testosterone
3. when an individual is excessively obese
4. when anticoagulants are administered in large doses
5. when calorie intake is diminished

7.23 Antiglobulins are involved in the:
1. Wassermann reaction
2. Coombs test
3. fluorescent antibody test
4. rheumatoid factor test
5. Casoni test

18.1   **Phaeochromocytoma may be associated with:**
1. paroxysmal hypertension
2. sweating
3. neurofibromatosis
4. a fall in blood pressure on palpating the abdomen
5. paroxysmal hypotension

12.3   **The common causes of cirrhosis of the liver in Great Britain are:**
1. alcohol
2. drugs such as halothane and paracetamol
3. hepatitis B
4. haemochromatosis
5. primary biliary cirrhosis

3.3   **Malignant disease may complicate the following chronic inflammatory diseases:**
1. chronic osteomyelitis
2. sarcoidosis
3. asbestosis
4. schistosomiasis
5. ulcerative colitis

7.36   **The following conditions are associated with T-cell immunodeficiency:**
1. Hodgkin's disease
2. Tay–Sachs disease
3. Wiskott–Aldrich syndrome
4. Down's syndrome
5. Di George syndrome

16.12   **Left-sided heart failure occurs as a complication of:**
1. hypertension
2. mitral regurgitation
3. pulmonary fibrosis
4. uncomplicated coronary atherosclerosis
5. tricuspid stenosis

6.10   **Ischaemic necrosis is a recognised complication of fractures of the following bones:**
1. talus
2. calcaneum
3. scaphoid
4. pisiform
5. femoral head

19.6   **The differences between the tubular lesions produced by nephrotoxic drugs and renal ischaemia include the following:**
1. the lesion produced by ischaemia occurs in a random fashion throughout all nephrons and in any part of the nephron down to collecting tubules
2. a nephrotoxic drug affects the entire nephron
3. nephrotoxic drugs produce scattered lesions throughout the kidney
4. ischaemia causes complete necrosis of the tubule cell together with the basement membrane
5. nephrotoxins cause both cytotoxic and ischaemic lesions

15.5   **The Epstein–Barr virus is associated with:**
1. glandular fever
2. the Australia antigen
3. Burkitt's lymphoma
4. nasopharyngeal carcinoma
5. the common cold

6.4   **Collagen, the ultimate source of the strength of a wound:**
1. is formed by undifferentiated mesenchymal cells
2. changes with the passage of time
3. undergoes lysis as well as synthesis even when the total collagen content of the wound is remaining constant
4. is broken down by the enzyme collagenase
5. is normally embedded in ground substance

4.10   **The incidence of postoperative infection can be reduced by the use of the following measures:**
1. the use of negative pressure ventilation in the operating theatre
2. the use of filtered air in the operating theatre, pore size 10 μm
3. showering by the surgeon and all attendants prior to embarking upon the operation
4. the administration of prophylactic antibiotics
5. disinfection of the patient's skin prior to operation

7.21 **An autoimmune haemolytic anaemia:**
1. does not occur in systemic lupus erythematosus
2. does not show Rhesus specificity
3. is associated with a negative Coombs test
4. may be caused by drug therapy
5. is not associated with leucopenia

22.3 **Ionising radiation:**
1. does not affect the eyes
2. affects renal function
3. does not affect the lungs
4. affects the brain
5. does not affect the skin

1.6 **Metaplasia, the transformation of one fully differentiated tissue into another, occurs in:**
1. connective tissue elements
2. the gastrointestinal tract
3. the central nervous system
4. the biliary system
5. the urothelium

7.12 **Active immunity can be produced by an appropriate vaccine to the following diseases:**
1. pneumococcal pneumonia
2. plague
3. chicken pox
4. poliomyelitis
5. typhoid

PAPER 10

Question number	Answer				
23.15	1. T	2. T	3. F	4. F	5. F
7.5	1. T	2. F	3. T	4. T	5. F
7.37	1. F	2. T	3. T	4. T	5. F
13.2	1. F	2. T	3. T	4. T	5. F
12.6	1. T	2. F	3. T	4. F	5. F
7.23	1. F	2. T	3. T	4. T	5. F
18.1	1. T	2. T	3. T	4. F	5. T
12.3	1. T	2. F	3. T	4. F	5. F
3.3	1. T	2. F	3. T	4. T	5. T
7.36	1. T	2. F	3. T	4. F	5. T
16.12	1. T	2. T	3. F	4. T	5. F
6.10	1. T	2. F	3. T	4. F	5. T
19.6	1. T	2. F	3. F	4. T	5. T
15.5	1. T	2. F	3. T	4. T	5. F
6.4	1. F	2. T	3. T	4. T	5. T
4.10	1. F	2. F	3. F	4. T	5. T
7.21	1. F	2. F	3. F	4. T	5. F
22.3	1. F	2. T	3. F	4. T	5. F
1.6	1. T	2. T	3. F	4. T	5. T
7.12	1. T	2. T	3. F	4. T	5. T

PAPER 11

23.16 Renal transplantation may be followed by:
1. infection
2. malignant neoplasia
3. amyloidosis
4. rheumatoid arthritis
5. psoriasis

7.32 The following substances are lymphokines:
1. properdin
2. migration inhibitory factor
3. macrophage chemotactic factor
4. factor B
5. interferon

16.8 Acquired syphilis of the cardiovascular system may involve the following lesions:
1. myocardial gummata
2. aortitis
3. aortic regurgitation
4. abdominal aortic aneurysm
5. stenosis of the coronary ostia

5.2 Spores are killed by exposure to:
1. moist heat at 110°C for 15 minutes
2. dry heat at 160°C for 1 hour
3. ethylene oxide
4. hydrogen peroxide
5. gentian violet

15.8 The following viral infections are controlled by cell-mediated immunity:
1. herpes simplex
2. cytomegalic inclusion disease
3. poliomyelitis
4. ECHO virus
5. vaccinia

18.9 The following tumours of the ovary secrete hormones:
1. arrhenoblastoma
2. dysgerminoma
3. dermoid cysts
4. papillary cystadenoma
5. granulosa-theca cell tumour

19.3   In renal tubular acidosis the following biochemical abnormalities occur:
1. an inability to lower the urine pH
2. abnormal ammonia excretion in relation to urine pH
3. renal glycosuria
4. hypercalciuria
5. hyperkalaemia

17.33   Platelets contribute to haemostasis by liberating:
1. 5-hydroxytryptamine (serotonin)
2. phospholipids
3. plasminogen
4. bradykinin
5. calcitonin

5.5   The following antibiotics are effective against fungi:
1. nystatin
2. bacitracin
3. griseofulvin
4. polymyxin B
5. amphotericin B

7.28   Cell-mediated immune processes are of great importance in the control of the following infections:
1. pneumococcal pneumonia
2. diphtheria
3. tuberculosis
4. candidiasis
5. mumps

19.8   Haemoglobinuria occurs:
1. in blackwater fever
2. following the excessive ingestion of beetroot
3. following extensive superficial burns
4. in blood transfusion
5. in strenuous exercise

21.6   Haemolytic disease of the newborn:
1. may be caused by *Treponema pallidum*
2. may be due to anti-c
3. may occur in the first pregnancy
4. frequently is not found until the second pregnancy
5. can be treated with anti-D antibodies

22.1   Ionising radiation:
1. increases DNA synthesis
2. increases H_2O_2 in the tissues
3. breaks disulphide bonds
4. causes atrophy of the seminiferous tubules of the testis
5. causes pathological fractures

18.6   Primary hyperparathyroidism is associated with:
1. bone cysts
2. carcinoma of the parathyroid glands
3. dystrophic calcification
4. hypertension
5. anorexia

8.5   The following conditions are associated with a polyclonal gammopathy:
1. Waldenström's macroglobulinaemia
2. rheumatoid arthritis
3. Down's syndrome
4. Wiskott–Aldrich syndrome
5. post-streptococcal glomerulonephritis

10.2   Angioneurotic oedema is associated with:
1. depression
2. complement deficiency
3. immunoglobulin E
4. menstruation
5. NSAID poisoning

14.4   General phenomena associated with neoplasia may include:
1. fever
2. cachexia
3. thrombotic episodes
4. polycythaemia
5. dermatomyositis

19.5   Acute tubular necrosis of the kidney commonly follows:
1. severe dehydration
2. the overadministration of carbon tetrachloride
3. acute porphyria
4. the overadministration of potassium chloride
5. gentamicin

17.6   Pathological destruction of red blood cells can take place in the following sites:
1. the submucosal plexus of the small intestine
2. the peripheral circulation
3. the liver
4. the spleen
5. the bone marrow

1.5   Starvation is associated with a reduction in size of the:
1. fat depots
2. heart
3. central nervous system
4. liver
5. bones

PAPER 11

Question number   *Answer*

23.16	1. T	2. T	3. F	4. F	5. F
7.32	1. F	2. T	3. T	4. F	5. T
16.8	1. T	2. T	3. T	4. F	5. T
5.2	1. F	2. T	3. T	4. F	5. F
15.8	1. T	2. T	3. F	4. F	5. T
18.9	1. T	2. F	3. T	4. F	5. T
19.3	1. T	2. F	3. F	4. T	5. F
17.33	1. T	2. T	3. F	4. F	5. F
5.5	1. T	2. F	3. T	4. F	5. T
7.28	1. F	2. F	3. T	4. T	5. T
19.8	1. T	2. F	3. F	4. F	5. T
21.6	1. F	2. T	3. T	4. T	5. T
22.1	1. F	2. T	3. F	4. T	5. T
18.6	1. T	2. T	3. F	4. T	5. T
8.5	1. F	2. T	3. F	4. F	5. T
10.2	1. F	2. F	3. T	4. F	5. F
14.4	1. T	2. T	3. T	4. T	5. T
19.5	1. T	2. T	3. T	4. F	5. F
17.6	1. F	2. T	3. T	4. T	5. T
1.5	1. T	2. T	3. F	4. T	5. F

PAPER 12

19.1   Renal function is depressed in the following conditions:
1. 'shock'
2. amyloidosis
3. chronic hyperuricaemia
4. irradiation
5. hypercalcaemia

14.8   Neuroblastoma are most common in:
1. children
2. may differentiate into benign tumours
3. the adrenal medulla
4. the floor of the fourth ventricle
5. sympathetic ganglia

7.20   Anaphylactic reactions commonly follow the administration of the following drugs:
1. penicillin
2. azathioprine
3. procaine
4. α-methyldopa
5. corticosteriods

24.8   Autosomal dominant diseases which are important to surgeons include:
1. hereditary spherocytosis
2. haemophilia
3. Von Recklinghausen's disease
4. familial agammaglobulinaemia
5. mucoviscidosis

8.2   The nephrotic syndrome is associated with:
1. no evidence of sodium retention
2. high levels of aldosterone in the urine
3. high levels of antidiuretic hormone in the urine
4. an increased blood volume
5. hypolipidaemia

2.5   the magnitude of the exudate associated with acute inflammation depends upon:
1. changes in the endothelium of the capillaries and venules
2. lymphocyte activation
3. the osmotic pressure of the plasma proteins
4. the plasma Ca^{++} level
5. the plasma K^+ level

13.8   **An increase in the frequency of malignant disease occurs in the following conditions:**
1. following the long term administration of immunosuppressive agents
2. large bowel Crohn's disease
3. coeliac disease
4. ulcerative colitis
5. xeroderma pigmentosum

2.3   **Normally the features of acute inflammation include:**
1. vasoconstriction
2. vasodilatation
3. infarction
4. haemolysis
5. oedema

22.9   **DNA synthesis is inhibited by:**
1. prednisone
2. methane sulphonic acid
3. methotrexate
4. azathioprine
5. chloramphenicol

17.5   **The production of red blood cells is depressed by the following conditions:**
1. chronic renal failure
2. excessive administration of glucocorticoids
3. subacute rheumatic fever
4. myxoedema
5. disseminated breast cancer

1.4   **Post menopausal ovarian atrophy is associated with the following structural changes:**
1. stromal hyperplasia
2. loss of ovarian weight
3. a proportionate decrease in size of the medulla
4. disappearance of primordial follicles
5. persistence of the germinal epithelium

23.17   **Acute rejection of a renal allograft involves:**
1. cellular infiltration of the donor kidney
2. a humoral component
3. subacute vasculitis
4. polymorphonuclear infiltration of the graft
5. a fall in the serum creatinine

17.26   Disorders of clotting occur in association with:
1. vitamin A deficiency
2. vitamin K deficiency
3. hereditary angioneurotic oedema
4. haemophilia
5. obstructive jaundice

1.2   Hypertrophy is associated with:
1. an increase in the number of visible mitoses
2. an increase in the bulk of a tissue
3. an increase in the number of cells in an organ or tissue
4. an absolute decrease in interstitial tissue
5. an increase in functional capacity

16.9   Coarctation of the aorta is associated with:
1. a primary developmental anomaly of the third left aortic arch
2. the development of a collateral circulation to overcome the effects of the abnormality
3. a bicuspid aortic valve
4. hypertension
5. erosion of the upper borders of the ribs

15.10   The following diseases are caused by chlamydia:
1. yellow fever
2. lymphogranuloma venereum
3. mumps
4. psittacosis
5. herpes simplex

17.9   Congenital spherocytosis is a haemolytic disorder:
1. inherited as an autosomal recessive
2. associated with chronic anaemia
3. basically caused by a developmental defect of the red cell membrane
4. associated with massive enlargement of the spleen
5. in which the osmotic fragility of the red cell is diminished

21.3   The following refer to blood group antigens:
1. Lewis
2. Von Willebrand
3. Duffy
4. Turner
5. Kidd

5.6   Benzyl penicillin is:
1. bacteriostatic
2. destroyed by the enzyme penicillinase
3. insoluble in water
4. damaging to the nucleus of the bacterial cell
5. active against some viruses

21.8   The following antibodies may pass across the placenta:
1. anti A isohaemagglutinin
2. immune antiblood group A
3. anti D (Rhesus)
4. diphtheria antitoxin
5. rheumatoid factor

PAPER 12

Question number	Answer				
19.1	1. T	2. T	3. T	4. T	5. T
14.8	1. T	2. T	3. T	4. F	5. T
7.20	1. T	2. F	3. T	4. F	5. F
24.8	1. T	2. F	3. T	4. F	5. F
8.2	1. F	2. T	3. T	4. F	5. F
2.5	1. T	2. F	3. T	4. F	5. F
13.8	1. T	2. F	3. T	4. T	5. T
2.3	1. T	2. T	3. F	4. F	5. T
22.9	1. F	2. T	3. T	4. T	5. F
17.5	1. T	2. F	3. T	4. T	5. T
1.4	1. T	2. T	3. F	4. T	5. T
23.17	1. T	2. T	3. T	4. F	5. F
17.26	1. F	2. T	3. F	4. T	5. T
1.2	1. F	2. T	3. F	4. F	5. T
16.9	1. F	2. T	3. T	4. F	5. F
15.10	1. F	2. T	3. F	4. T	5. F
17.9	1. F	2. T	3. T	4. F	5. F
21.3	1. T	2. F	3. T	4. F	5. T
5.6	1. F	2. T	3. F	4. F	5. F
21.8	1. F	2. T	3. T	4. T	5. F

24.11   The glycogen storage diseases are associated with the following enzyme defects:
1. amylase
2. glucose-6-phosphatase
3. amylo, 1, 6-glucosidase
4. glutamic oxaloacetic transaminase
5. nucleotide adenophosphodehydrogenase

4.13   The common pathogenic pyogenic organisms affecting man include:
1. *Staphylococcus aureus*
2. *Clostridium tetani*
3. *Staphylococcus albus*
4. *Bacteroides*
5. *Pseudomonas aeruginosa*

17.24   The chief characteristics of Burkitt's lymphoma are that:
1. it is commonest in young adults
2. it is associated with the Epstein–Barr virus
3. it is uncommon In malarial areas
4. the commonest parts of the body involved are the facial bones and lower jaw
5. the characteristic cells of the tumour are poorly differentiated large lymphocytes and large pale histocytes

7.25   The following tests are based upon a delayed hypersensitivity reaction:
1. Schick test
2. Wassermann reaction
3. Frei test
4. Leishmanin test
5. Prausnitz–Kustner reaction

17.8   The following haemolytic disorders are congenital:
1. thalassaemia
2. March haemoglobinuria
3. microangiopathic haemolytic anaemia
4. ovalocytosis
5. G6PD deficiency

9.2   Hypercalcaemia is associated with:
1. increased excitability of the neuromuscular apparatus
2. band keratitis
3. metastatic calcification
4. prolonged Q–T interval
5. renal stones

17.27 The formation of a clot is affected by the following substances:
1. zinc
2. calcium
3. Factor B
4. Factor IX
5. kallikrein

12.10 The following biochemical disturbances occur in fulminating hepatic failure:
1. metabolic acidosis
2. prolongation of the prothrombin time
3. hyperglycaemia
4. hyperbilirubinaemia
5. low serum albumin

8.1 The total plasma protein level is low in:
1. patients suffering from protein-losing enteropathy
2. patients suffering from cardiac failure associated with oedema
3. oedema due to the nephrotic syndrome
4. nutritional oedema
5. patients suffering from chronic liver disease

17.30 Which of the following functions are carried out by platelets:
1. binding of antigen-antibody complexes
2. secretion of clotting factors
3. secretion of prostaglandins
4. release of the Hageman factor
5. release of vasoactive amines

24.13 Prostaglandins are:
1. formed from complement
2. vasodilators
3. involved in clotting
4. inhibited by azathioprine
5. inhibited by aspirin

17.21 Monocytic leukaemia, now more commonly known as Hairy Cell leukaemia:
1. is the commonest form of leukaemia
2. is associated with monocytes or monoblasts in the peripheral blood
3. may present with increasing anaemia
4. is associated with nodular infiltrative skin lesions
5. can present as an acute myelo-monocytic form

4.3   The following diseases are the result of arthropod-borne blood infections:
1. cholera
2. trypanosomiasis
3. tetanus
4. malaria
5. hydatid disease

23.18 HIV is:
1. a retrovirus
2. dependent on reverse transcriptase for its replication
3. causes a monoclonal hypergammaglobulaemia
4. associated with the production of excessive amounts of IgG2
5. related to T-cell leukaemia

24.12 A vaccine:
1. contains one or more antigens
2. produces active immunity
3. contains one or more antibodies
4. stimulates polymorphonuclear leucocyte activity
5. can be administered orally

4.12   Staphylococci pathogenic to man:
1. produce a capsular polysaccharide
2. grow in irregular clusters in culture
3. produce coagulase
4. are resistant to penicillin
5. all produce an enterotoxin

17.23 Hodgkin's lymphoma has recently been reclassified into four histological groups. Regardless of classification, however, which of the following cell types are found in the lymph nodes in this disease:
1. lymphocytes
2. basophils
3. eosinophils
4. Reed–Sternberg cells
5. polymorphonuclear leucocytes

13.9 **An enhancement of tumour growth or an increased incidence of tumour formation may occur:**
1. following the long term administration of immunosuppressive drugs
2. following immunological enhancement
3. due to the release of soluble antigens by the tumour cells
4. due to an alteration of T-cell function
5. due to the excessive production or release of lysosomal enzymes

17.4 **Iron deficiency anaemia may be associated with the following:**
1. a sensitive and painful glossitis
2. dysphagia
3. a rise in the liver iron
4. koilonychia
5. chlorosis

21.5 **The physical results of Rhesus incompatibility include the following:**
1. hydrops fetalis
2. Hutchinson's teeth
3. icterus neonatorum
4. hepato-lenticular degeneration
5. kernicterus

PAPER 13

Question number	Answer				
24.11	1. F	2. T	3. T	4. F	5. F
4.13	1. T	2. F	3. F	4. T	5. T
17.24	1. F	2. T	3. F	4. T	5. T
7.25	1. F	2. F	3. T	4. T	5. F
17.8	1. T	2. F	3. F	4. T	5. T
9.2	1. F	2. T	3. T	4. F	5. T
17.27	1. F	2. T	3. F	4. T	5. F
12.10	1. T	2. T	3. F	4. T	5. F
8.1	1. T	2. F	3. T	4. T	5. T
17.30	1. T	2. F	3. T	4. F	5. T
24.13	1. F	2. T	3. T	4. F	5. T
17.21	1. F	2. T	3. T	4. T	5. T
4.3	1. F	2. T	3. F	4. T	5. F
23.18	1. T	2. T	3. F	4. F	5. T
24.12	1. T	2. T	3. F	4. F	5. T
4.12	1. F	2. T	3. T	4. F	5. F
17.23	1. T	2. F	3. T	4. T	5. T
13.9	1. T	2. T	3. T	4. T	5. F
17.4	1. F	2. T	3. F	4. T	5. T
21.5	1. T	2. F	3. T	4. F	5. T

PAPER 14

17.15 **An absolute lymphocytosis occurs in the following conditions:**
1. extensive skin diseases such as psoriasis, eczema, pemphigus
2. Loeffler's syndrome
3. tuberculosis
4. pertussis
5. chronic lymphatic leukaemia

4.11 **Renal tract infection is caused by a variety of bacteria including:**
1. Streptococcus pyogenes
2. Klebsiella pneumoniae
3. Streptococcus faecalis
4. Staphylococcus aureus
5. Escherichia coli

8.3 **Secondary hypogammaglobulinaemia occurs in:**
1. sarcoidosis
2. congestive heart failure
3. malnutrition
4. chronic lymphatic leukaemia
5. nephrotic syndrome

12.5 **A diminution in the bile salt pool and hence a diminished concentration of bile salts in the bile occurs:**
1. in jejunal diverticulosis
2. in diseases affecting the terminal ileum such as Crohn's disease
3. due to the eating of refined carbohydrates
4. in ulcerative colitis
5. in congenital deficiency of cholesterol 7α-hydroxylase

17.1 **A low mean corpuscular haemoglobin concentration occurs in the following:**
1. iron deficiency anaemia
2. pernicious anaemia
3. the anaemia associated with infestation with the fish tapeworm *Diphyllobothrium latum*
4. the anaemia following extensive gastric resection
5. sideroblastic anaemia

18.2 **Increased amounts of erythropoietin are found in the plasma:**
1. in pernicious anaemia
2. in iron deficiency anaemia
3. following bleeding
4. in erythroblastosis foetalis
5. in kwashiorkor

17.3   The following are haemoglobinopathies:
1. congenital spherocytosis
2. sickle-cell anaemia
3. thalassaemia
4. cold agglutination immune haemolytic anaemia
5. eliptocystosis

4.4   *Streptococcus faecalis:*
1. is a common inhabitant of the gastrointestinal tract
2. grows in long chains
3. flourishes in bile-salt lactose media
4. is concerned in the aetiology of periodontal disease
5. is an opportunistic rather than a true pathogen

13.11   The incidence of tumours is increased in:
1. sarcoidosis
2. Wiskott–Aldrich syndrome
3. ataxia telangiectasis
4. patients treated over long periods with corticosteroids
5. patients receiving azathioprine

17.17   Myeloid metaplasia is associated with:
1. a variable peripheral white count
2. extramedullary haemopoiesis
3. the Philadelphia chromosome
4. a decreased number of megakaryocytes in the marrow
5. anaemia

14.11   The 'doubling time' of a malignant tumour is affected by a number of factors including:
1. a decrease in cell cycle time
2. exfoliation
3. the percentage of cells in the resting phase
4. the oxygen content of the tumour cell's environment
5. nuclear size

17.16   Acute myeloblastic leukaemia:
1. is most common in young adults
2. is associated with the presence of a large number of primitive cells in the marrow and peripheral blood
3. is associated with peripheral white counts in excess of 100 000 per μl
4. may be associated with a normal white count
5. marrow aspirates show decreased cellularity

8.4   A monoclonal gammopathy occurs in the following diseases:
1. lepromatous leprosy
2. kala-azar
3. multiple myeloma
4. lymphatic leukaemia
5. active chronic hepatitis

11.4   Hereditary or idiopathic haemochromatosis is:
1. more common in the female than the male
2. an autosomal recessive disorder
3. associated with a material staining with Congo Red
4. complicated by malignancy
5. associated with arthritis

13.3   The following pathological conditions can be regarded as precancerous:
1. osteitis deformans
2. leukoplakia
3. fibroadenosis of the breast
4. duodenal ulceration
5. cervical erosions

16.7   The investigations performed in a patient suffering from Raynaud's phenomenon should include:
1. assay of haemagglutinating antibodies
2. rheumatoid factor
3. antimitochondrial antibodies
4. serum potassium
5. X-ray of the root of the neck

10.1   Oedema occurs in:
1. Cushing's syndrome
2. Conn's Syndrome
3. Zollinger–Ellison syndrome
4. Klinefelter's syndrome
5. pregnancy

14.2   Broder's classification of tumours attempted to classify tumours according to:
1. their origin
2. the degree of differentiation of a tumour
3. the degree of stromal response
4. the degree of lymphocytic infiltration of the tumour
5. the number of mitoses found in a given area of the tumour

16.13   A myocardial infarct may be associated with:
1. hypotension
2. a fall in the plasma GOT
3. endocardial thrombosis
4. a red infarct
5. atrial rather than ventricular fibrillation

15.9   Interferons:
1. are cytokines
2. can be produced in response to mitogens
3. are components of the complement system
4. are important in viral infections
5. are a dialysable fraction

11.3   The following endocrine abnormalities lead to generalized pigmentation:
1. Cushing's disease
2. carcinoid tumours
3. Zollinger–Ellison syndrome
4. Addison's disease
5. Sheehan's syndrome

PAPER 14

Question number	Answer				
17.15	1. F	2. F	3. T	4. T	5. T
4.11	1. F	2. T	3. T	4. T	5. T
8.3	1. F	2. F	3. T	4. T	5. T
12.5	1. F	2. T	3. T	4. F	5. T
17.1	1. T	2. F	3. F	4. T	5. F
18.2	1. T	2. T	3. T	4. T	5. F
17.3	1. F	2. T	3. T	4. F	5. F
4.4	1. T	2. F	3. T	4. T	5. T
13.11	1. F	2. T	3. T	4. F	5. T
17.17	1. T	2. T	3. F	4. F	5. T
14.11	1. F	2. T	3. T	4. T	5. F
17.16	1. F	2. T	3. F	4. T	5. F
8.4	1. F	2. F	3. T	4. T	5. F
11.4	1. F	2. T	3. F	4. T	5. T
13.3	1. T	2. T	3. F	4. F	5. F
16.7	1. T	2. T	3. F	4. F	5. T
10.1	1. T	2. F	3. F	4. F	5. T
14.2	1. F	2. T	3. F	4. F	5. T
16.13	1. T	2. F	3. T	4. F	5. F
15.9	1. T	2. F	3. F	4. T	5. F
11.3	1. T	2. F	3. F	4. T	5. F

PAPER 15

16.6   Liquefaction associated with necrosis occurs after infarction of the:
1. heart
2. kidney
3. brain
4. liver
5. spleen

7.30   Which of the following tests may be used to assess host resistance to mycobacterial infections:
1. skin tests
2. complement fixation
3. lymphocyte transformation test
4. radio immunoassay
5. leucocyte migration inhibition test

10.7   The essential constituents of primary amyloid include:
1. immunoglobulin
2. complement
3. albumin
4. starch
5. fibrils

6.6   The following are the features associated with the healing of open wounds:
1. the formation of granulation tissue
2. infection
3. migration of the surrounding epithelium
4. giant cell formation
5. contraction

20.5   Combined water and electrolyte depletion causes:
1. a high concentration of sodium in the urine
2. a high urine specific gravity
3. pre-renal uraemia
4. a fall in the central venous pressure
5. a high blood urea nitrogen to creatinine ratio

15.1   The following are viral diseases:
1. cytomegalic inclusion disease
2. trachoma
3. dengue
4. primary atypical pneumonia
5. typhus

17.31   Thrombocytopenia can be caused by:
1. deficiency of clotting factors
2. haemorrhage
3. diuretics
4. measles virus
5. telangiectasia

13.4   The following are carcinogenic:
1. infra-red radiation
2. ultra-violet radiation
3. house dust
4. soot
5. mould

18.3   An eosinophil adenoma of the anterior hypophysis is associated with:
1. enlargement of the sella turcica
2. hypertrophy and hyperplasia of the soft tissues throughout the body
3. excessive growth of the acral parts
4. premature closure of the epiphyses
5. impaired glucose tolerance

2.4   The blood flow through acutely inflamed tissues is decreased by the following events:
1. increased cellular concentration in the blood flowing through the inflamed part
2. loss of protein from the dilated capillaries
3. aggregation of the red cells
4. adherence of leucocytes to the capillary endothelium
5. Lewis' axon reflex

3.8   Direct evidence of immunological activity can be demonstrated in the following chronic inflammatory diseases:
1. lepromatous leprosy
2. tuberculoid leprosy
3. silicosis
4. rheumatoid arthritis
5. asbestosis

4.6   Bacteria are normally found on or in the:
1. blood
2. urinary tract
3. lower bronchi
4. gastrointestinal tract
5. skin, sebaceous glands and hair follicles

9.5   Excessive osteoid tissue is found in:
1. vitamin D deficiency
2. Muslim women
3. patients on anticonvulsant drugs
4. patients on long-term anticoagulant therapy
5. long-standing obstructive jaundice

12.7   The main constituents of gall stones are:
1. calcium sulphate
2. cholesterol
3. calcium palmitate
4. calcium bilirubinate
5. amorphous materials

20.4   The blood urea is elevated in the following conditions:
1. severe dehydration
2. pregnancy
3. tubular necrosis
4. diabetes insipidus
5. cortical necrosis

6.3   The healing of a wound is delayed by:
1. vitamin C deficiency
2. starvation
3. the administration of glucocorticoids
4. lack of blood supply
5. infection

4.1   Infection within a hospital may be:
1. dust-borne
2. water-borne
3. food-borne
4. hand-borne
5. endogenous

21.2   The following tests should be performed on donor blood before it is used for transfusion:
1. HBsAg
2. Van den Bergh
3. Wassermann test or the VDRL flocculation test
4. acid phosphatase
5. malaria smear

PAPER 15

Question number	Answer				
16.6	1. F	2. F	3. T	4. F	5. F
7.30	1. T	2. F	3. T	4. F	5. T
10.7	1. T	2. F	3. F	4. F	5. T
6.6	1. T	2. T	3. T	4. F	5. T
20.5	1. F	2. T	3. T	4. T	5. F
15.1	1. T	2. F	3. T	4. F	5. F
17.31	1. F	2. T	3. T	4. T	5. F
13.4	1. F	2. T	3. F	4. T	5. T
18.3	1. T	2. T	3. T	4. F	5. T
2.4	1. T	2. F	3. T	4. T	5. F
3.8	1. F	2. T	3. F	4. T	5. F
4.6	1. F	2. F	3. F	4. T	5. T
9.5	1. T	2. T	3. T	4. F	5. T
12.7	1. F	2. T	3. T	4. T	5. T
20.4	1. T	2. F	3. T	4. F	5. T
6.3	1. T	2. T	3. T	4. T	5. T
4.1	1. T	2. T	3. T	4. T	5. T
21.2	1. T	2. F	3. T	4. F	5. T

Part 2: Questions and answers with explanations

1.1 Disuse atrophy follows:
  1. blockage of the duct of an exocrine gland
  2. immobilisation of a joint
  3. interference with the nerve supply to the muscles controlling joint movement
  4. interference with the blood supply
  5. the diminished secretion of trophic hormones

1. True
An excellent example is the pancreas. Ligation of the main pancreatic duct leads to atrophy of the exocrine portion of the gland but the endocrine portion, i.e. islets of Langerhans, continue to function normally.

2. True
Immobilisation of the knee provides a good example. An internal derangement of this joint, such as damage to a cartilage, is rapidly followed by atrophy of the quadriceps group of muscles, especially of vastus medialis.

3. False
Interruption of the nerve supply to a group of muscles causes a specific neuropathic atrophy in the affected group of muscles. However, the bone to which such muscles are attached may undergo true atrophy due simply to inactivity if the condition is irreversible, e.g. anterior poliomyelitis.

4. False
Reduction of the blood supply to a tissue causes atrophy due to defective nutrition.

5. False
The diminished secretion of trophic hormones such as T_4 by the thyroid does produce atrophic changes in target organs such as the skin, hair follicles, sweat gland and sebaceous glands but this is not disuse atrophy. These changes can be readily reversed by the administration of thyroxine.

1.2 Hypertrophy is associated with:
  1. an increase in the number of visible mitoses
  2. an increase in the bulk of a tissue

3. an increase in the number of cells in an organ or tissue
4. an absolute decrease in interstitial tissue
5. an increase in functional capacity

1. False
In pure hypertrophy the number of cells remains the same in contrast to hyperplasia in which the number of cells increases. No evidence of excessive mitoses is, therefore, normally seen.

2. True
This is the chief change in hypertrophy. It is seen to best advantage in the hypertrophied muscles of an athlete or in the cardiac muscle in response to hypertension, aortic stenosis or regurgitation.

3. False
Pure hypertrophy is not associated with an increase in the number of cells but only with an increase in the size of those already present.

4. False
The volume of interstitial tissue does not alter. Any apparent decrease is relative, produced by the enlargement of the specialised cells of the organ or tissue.

5. True
The functional capacity of all organs and tissues in which hypertrophy occurs is increased. For example, the increased thickness and length of hypertrophied muscles leads to increased power. Another example is the hypertrophy of the remaining kidney following unilateral nephrectomy. The remaining kidney, if this is normal, increases in size and functional capacity. In part this is due to true hypertrophy but in addition hyperplasia also occurs with an increase in the number of component cells of the glomeruli and tubules.

1.3   Old age is specifically associated with atrophic changes in:
1. bone
2. the kidneys
3. the bone marrow
4. the brain
5. the ovaries

1. True
The radiological density of bone progressively decreases in both men and women with advancing age. This change is indistinguishable from osteoporosis, in which condition the amount of uncalcified bone may become so great that bone pain and fractures may occur.

2. True
Increasing age is associated with a gradual loss in the number of nephrons and a gradual reduction in renal functional capacity. At

ninety years of age the overall function of kidneys has diminished by about 50%. The decrease of glomerular filtration is particularly important in relation to the administration of drugs such as digitalis and some antibiotics.

3. True
Gradual replacement of the red marrow takes place with advancing age.

4. True
Old age is associated with loss of neurons and neuroglial overgrowth causing senile or presenile dementia. These changes occur more rapidly in the presence of ischaemia.

5. True
Ovarian atrophy is associated with a decline in weight of these organs from approximately 14 g to around 5 g in the sixth decade. The primordial follicles largely disappear and marked stromal hyperplasia occurs.

1.4 **Post menopausal ovarian atrophy is associated with the following structural changes:**
1. stromal hyperplasia
2. loss of ovarian weight
3. a proportionate decrease in size of the medulla
4. disappearance of primordial follicles
5. persistence of the germinal epithelium

1. True
Marked stromal hyperplasia occurs after 40 years of age, possibly due to continued hormone production by the ovaries.

2. True
The weight of the premenopausal ovary is about 14 g; by the fifth, sixth and seventh decades it falls to 5 g.

3. False
Relative to the cortex the medullary portion of the ovary, in which the corpora albicantia are situated, is proportionately larger in the post menopausal ovary. In both areas the stromal elements become fibrotic.

4. True
Rarely a few immature follicles undergoing maturation and atresia may be seen in the corticomedullary junction in the first five years after the menopause.

5. True
The germinal epithelium persists and follows the various convolutions on the surface but in some places, this intimate connection with the surface may be lost and small cysts may form.

1.5   Starvation is associated with a reduction in size of the:
1. fat depots
2. heart
3. central nervous system
4. liver
5. bones

In the first phase of starvation the fat depots disappear and this is later followed by a gradual reduction in the size of organs such as the gastrointestinal tract, liver and heart while the central nervous system and skeleton remain unaffected. The correct answers are, therefore,

1. **True**
2. **True**
3. **False**
4. **True**
5. **False**

An exception to this general pattern occurs in kwashiorkor. In this condition, which affects infants and young children in many parts of Southern and Central Africa and the Far East, the diet is deficient in high grade protein but moderately adequate in total calories due to a high carbohydrate intake. Growth is impaired. The liver is enlarged because of fatty infiltration but depleted of RNA and protein.

1.6   Metaplasia, the transformation of one fully differentiated tissue into another, occurs in:
1. connective tissue elements
2. the gastrointestinal tract
3. the central nervous system
4. the biliary system
5. the urothelium

1. True
True bone may occasionally develop in an operation scar.

2. True
Metaplasia occurs in some parts of the gastrointestinal tract under abnormal circumstances. A common site is in the mucus secreting columnar epithelium of the anal canal. When this mucosa prolapses through the anal sphincter, as in third degree haemorrhoids or a true rectal prolapse, the resulting chronic irritation results in a change to squamous epithelium.

3. False
No metaplastic changes occur in the central nervous system.

4. True
Metaplasia of the gall bladder epithelium occurs in cholelithiasis. Such change may be eventually followed by the development of a squamous cell carcinoma because of a change from tall columnar to a squamous type of epithelium.

5. True

Epithelial metaplasia is usually associated with a change to a less specialized or complex type of epithelium. The urothelium is an important exception. In the bladder the presence of chronic inflammation (excluding tuberculosis) leads to cystitis cystica. The transitional epithelium grows downwards in solid clumps into the submucosa and if these become detached a central space may develop and since these cells may acquire mucus-secreting properties the end result is a glandular mucous membrane.

A similar process in the ureters leads to the condition of ureteritis cystitis. Calculi in the urinary tract cause the normal transitional epithelium over a period to become squamous in type, a change which may be followed by the development of a squamous carcinoma.

SECTION 2. ACUTE INFLAMMATION

2.1 Acute inflammation can be caused by:
1. *Streptococcus pneumoniae*
2. *Mycobacterium tuberculosis*
3. *Neisseria meningitidis*
4. *Mycobacterium leprae*
5. *Borrelia vincenti*

1. True

Streptococcus pneumoniae is the causal organism of lobar pneumonia.

2. True

Although *Mycobacterium tuberculosis* is more commonly associated with 'chronic' inflammation, acute tuberculous inflammation does occur particularly following infection of the meninges or pleura.

3. True

Neisseria meningitidis is the causal organism of acute meningitis, a disease once referred to as 'spotted fever' because in the presence of meningococcal septicaemia a haemorrhagic rash occurs.

4. False

Mycobacterium leprae is never associated with acute inflammation. Two forms of leprosy occur, lepromatous and tuberculoid.

5. True

Borrelia vincenti is the causal agent of Vincent's angina, an acute inflammation of the gums and oropharynx. The organism itself is an anaerobic flexuous spirochaete with three to eight irregular coils. It is a normal commensal in the mouth.

2.2   The following agents produce an acute inflammatory reaction in unsensitised individuals:
1. lipopolysaccharide
2. albumin
3. ultraviolet light
4. insulin
5. carbon particles

1. True
Lipopolysaccharides are the chemical structure of bacterial endotoxins. An immediate acute inflammatory reaction occurs following an intradermal injection of an endotoxin. If a subsequent intravenous injection of polysaccharide is administered some 24 hours later a local haemorrhagic reaction associated with tissue necrosis at the site of the previous intradermal injection occurs. (Schwartzmann reaction)

2. False
An intradermal injection of albumin does not cause an inflammatory reaction unless an individual has been previously sensitised.

3. True
Radiation injury which may be due to heat or ionising radiation in addition to ultraviolet light can cause an acute inflammatory reaction. The initial reaction is the triple response which follows histamine release.

4. False
Insulin does not cause an inflammatory reaction in unsensitised individuals.

5. False
Carbon particles are biologically inactive although some of the carbon which is inhaled is engulfed by macrophages and is retained within the relatively immobile alveoli adjacent to the bronchioles, blood vessels and fibrous septa producing the blackening which is seen in nearly every adult lung of city dwellers at autopsy.

2.3   Normally the features of acute inflammation include:
1. vasoconstriction
2. vasodilatation
3. infarction
4. haemolysis
5. oedema

1. True
The earliest change following the initiation of acute inflammation is constriction of small blood vessels.

2. True
The initial capillary constriction is rapidly followed by vasodilatation. This gives rise to the first part of the triple response described by

Lewis, the 'red line'. This, in turn, is followed by arteriolar dilatation producing the 'flare' after which increased permeability of the small blood vessels causes the appearance of a 'weal'. This triple response can be readily reproduced by pricking histamine into the skin and can be blocked by antihistamines. It is, however, probably of little practical importance in acute bacterial inflammation.

3. False
Infarction is commonly due to the obstruction of an end artery, usually by an embolus. This causes a segmental area of tissue necrosis and whilst the necrotic area itself does not become inflamed the surrounding tissues show all the histological changes associated with inflammation.

4. False
The intravascular lysis of erythrocytes does not normally accompany acute inflammation. It may, however, develop due to the liberation of exotoxins by the infecting organisms, such as *Clostridium welchii* and *Streptococcus pyogenes*.

5. True
The exudation of fluid from the blood vessels in an inflamed area gives rise to swelling which is one of the cardinal signs of inflammation. The exudate is caused by several factors, including:
  (a) the hydrostatic pressure in the small blood vessels exceeding the osmotic pressure of the plasma proteins
  (b) an increase in small vessel permeability caused by the chemical mediators of inflammation
  (c) an inability of the lymphatics to remove the increased quantities of interstitial fluid.

2.4 The blood flow through acutely inflamed tissues is decreased by the following events:
  1. increased cellular concentration in the blood flowing through the inflamed part
  2. loss of protein from the dilated capillaries
  3. aggregation of the red cells
  4. adherence of leucocytes to the capillary endothelium
  5. Lewis' axon reflex

1. True
The cellular concentration of the blood in the capillaries and post-capillary venules of an inflamed tissue is increased. This occurs because as fluid escapes from the dilated blood vessels due to their increased permeability, the cellular concentration automatically increases and as a result causes an increase in blood viscosity.

2. False
Although protein loss does occur the fluid loss is greater, causing an elevation in the plasma protein concentration and hence an increase in viscosity.

3. True
The red cells aggregate into rouleaux which lead to sludging, a process first described by Kniseley. This further increases the viscosity of the blood.

4. True
The effective lumen of the post-capillary venules is greatly reduced by the adherence of the leucocytes to one another and to the endothelium of the capillaries and post-capillary venules.

5. False
It is doubtful whether the axon reflex is of any practical importance in the acute inflammatory process.

2.5   The magnitude of the exudate associated with acute inflammation depends upon:
1. changes in the endothelium of the capillaries and venules
2. lymphocyte activation
3. the osmotic pressure of the plasma proteins
4. the plasma Ca^{++} level
5. the plasma K^+ level

1. True
A number of chemical mediators act on the capillary endothelium to increase its permeability thus allowing the escape of protein rich fluid into the area of acute inflammation. Among these various chemicals are histamine, a variety of kinins, prostaglandins and a number of complement components.

2. False
There is no evidence that lymphocyte activation, which is important in cell-mediated immune reactions, delayed hypersensitivity and chronic inflammation, plays a major role in acute inflammation.

3. True
The osmotic pressure of the plasma and the inflammatory exudate is dependent upon the protein concentration. When the osmotic pressure in the exudate is higher than in the vessels, more fluid will be drawn from the vessels into the exudate.

4. False
There is no evidence, as yet, that plasma Ca^{++} levels affect the acute inflammatory response although the concentration of calcium does, however, play an important role in intracellular events. Thus the movement of extracellular calcium into the cell can activate a number of events through cyclic nucleotides.

5. False
There is no evidence that potassium concentration plays any part in the local inflammatory response. Hypo- or hyperkalaemia does, however, have important physiological effects, particularly on the myocardium.

2.6   The following cell types are involved in acute inflammation:
1. polymorphonuclear leucocytes
2. lymphocytes
3. endothelial cells
4. epithelioid cells
5. mast cells

1. True
The polymorphonuclear leucocyte is the chief cell involved in the acute inflammatory reaction. In a normal blood stream the leucocytes are confined to the central axial column, but as the blood flow slows as a result of increased vascular permeability, the white cells fall out of the central column and become marginated, so that in due course the capillary endothelium is paved with such cells. At this point, by inserting pseudopods between the endothelial cells, the polymorphs first squeeze between the endothelial cells and then the basement membrane to reach the extravascular space, after which they migrate towards the site of injury under the influence of chemotaxis. These processes are governed by a variety of chemical mediators. Migration is under the influence of a large number of adhesion receptors and chemotaxis is governed by a number of exogenous and endogenous substances which act as chemoattractants. The commonest exogenous attractants are the bacteria themselves and the endogenous mediators include components of the complement system especially C5, leukotrienes, especially B4, and cytokines chiefly IL8.

2. False
Lymphocytes play no major role in the early stages of acute inflammation. They are, however, of greater importance in chronic inflammation and are particularly important in those inflammatory processes which involve cell-mediated immunity.

3. True
Changes in the endothelium result in an increase in capillary permeability and the adherence of polymorphonuclear leucocytes to the walls of small blood vessels. Such changes are probably brought about by chemical mediators among which histamine, bradykinin and the prostaglandins appear to be important.

4. False
Epithelioid cells which are derived from mononuclear phagocyte cells are not seen in acute inflammation. They are associated with long standing chronic inflammation and are seen in the centre of granulomas caused by such agents are *Mycobacterium tuberculosis.*

5. True
Mast cells secrete histamine, serotonin, SRS-A and kallikrein, all of which play a role in the acute inflammatory process. Degranulation of the mast cells is an important step in the release of histamine from these cells, this chemical agent being one of the earliest chemical mediators found in acutely inflamed tissues.

2.7   **The magnitude of leucocyte migration into an area infected with bacteria is governed by:**
1. the type of organism causing the inflammatory lesion
2. chemotaxins
3. the C5a complement component
4. the phosphatase levels in the inflamed area
5. the formation of pus

1. True
The intensity of the leucocytic infiltration into an infected lesion varies considerably. Some bacteria, notably the pyogenic organisms, such as *Streptococcus pyogenes*, *Staphylococcus aureus* and *Streptococcus pneumoniae* are associated with an intense leucocytic infiltration. Others such as *Salmonella typhi* and *Clostridium welchii*, although causing severe inflammation, do not provoke a severe degree of leucocytic infiltration.

2. True
Chemotaxins are chemical substances which stimulate migration of the leucocytes in a particular direction. Identifiable chemotaxins include bacterial products, lysates of the polymorphonuclear cells and extracts from the inflamed tissues.

3. True
C5a is a product of reacted complement. In certain circumstances it can be shown that complement depletion is associated with a decrease in leucocyte migration into an inflamed area.

4. False
Phosphatase levels play no part in the acute inflammatory process.

5. True
Lysates of the polymorphonuclear cells are very potent chemotactic agents when incubated with serum and it can, therefore, be assumed that pus formation increases leucocyte migration.

2.8   **The main components of the pyogenic membrane are:**
1. eosinophils
2. capillary loops
3. hyaluronidase
4. polymorphonuclear leucocytes
5. fibroblasts

1. False
Eosinophil cells play no part in the acute inflammatory response which normally initiates the formation of a pyogenic membrane.

2. True
The proliferation of capillary loops is a characteristic feature of granulation tissue. When the original factor initiating the formation of the membrane, e.g. the pyogenic organism, has been eliminated

either by the body's natural defence mechanisms or by the administration of antibiotics the capillary loops grow into the inflamed zone at up to 2 mm a day supported by ground substance.

3. False
Hyaluronidase is an enzyme produced by some bacteria such as the clostridia, the organisms responsible for gas gangrene. By destroying the connective tissue ground substance, it enables organisms to spread along tissue planes.

4. True
Polymorphonuclear leucocytes migrate into the ground substance from the capillary loop in order to phagocytose bacteria. Peripheral to these cells may be plasma cells, lymphocytes and macrophages, all cells concerned with the natural defence mechanisms.

5. True
Fibroblasts accompany the capillary loops and are dependent upon them for their oxygen supply. When the acute inflammatory reaction falters and the stage of healing has been reached, the fibroblasts lay down collagen.

2.9 The following are the chemical mediators involved in acute inflammation:
1. complement
2. histamine
3. insulin
4. bradykinin
5. lymphokine

1. True
The C3a and C5a components of complement are powerful chemotactic agents attracting polymorphonuclear leucocytes to a site of acute inflammation. In addition these compounds also act as anaphylatoxins causing histamine release from the mast cells with the result that plain muscle contracts and vasoconstriction follows.

2. True
Histamine liberated by the degranulation of mast cells is one of the most important causes of the changes seen in the early phase of acute inflammation, a phase which can be markedly depressed by the administration of antihistamines.

3. False
This substance plays no known role in acute inflammation. It is secreted by the β cells of the islets of Langerhans and is a major factor in controlling the circulating level of glucose. An increase in its secretion causes an enhanced uptake of glucose by the hepatocytes and a decrease in glucose absorption from the intestine.

4. True
Bradykinin is a nonapeptide derived from a plasma euglobulin by the digestion of the latter by proteolytic enzymes. Among these are

kallikrein which is present in the plasma as an inactive precursor which is activated by the Hageman factor. Bradykinin causes pain, erythema and increased vascular permeability and hence swelling of an acutely inflamed area.

5. False
Lymphokines are not concerned with acute inflammation but are considered to be the mediators of delayed hypersensitivity. They are secreted by lymphocytes which have been activated by a specific antigen or mitogen. They are chemotactic to mononuclear cells, inhibit the migration of macrophages in vitro and cause delayed inflammatory reactions in the skin.

2.10   The following substances are involved in acute inflammation:
   1. peptides
   2. lectins
   3. plasmin
   4. LATS
   5. PGE_1

1. True
Peptides composed of between 8 and 14 amino acid residues increase vascular permeability and hence increase the volume of exudate accompanying an acute inflammatory reaction. Such peptides are derived from protein in the exudate by the action of proteolytic enzymes derived from the plasma, tissue cells and polymorphonuclear leucocytes.

2. True
Lectins are a group of transmembrane molecules belonging to the wider group known as selectins which are concerned with cellular adhesion. Hence they are an important part of the mechanism by which polymorphonuclear leucocytes adhere to the capillary endothelium, which is a necessary step prior to their migration into the extravascular space.

3. True
Plasmin is intimately concerned with the acute inflammatory response. It is a proteolytic enzyme produced from the plasma plasminogen by the action of activators such as urokinase and streptokinase. Among the various actions of plasmin is its ability to break down fibrin to soluble degradation products, hence the use of activators in thrombolytic therapy. In addition it splits kininogen to form bradykinin and acts on the C3 component of complement to produce C3a and C3b. The former is a strong chemotactic agent and anaphylatoxin and the latter promote phagocytosis.

4. False
LATS, long acting thyroid stimulator is not involved in acute inflammation.

5. True
This substance causes vasodilatation, increases capillary permeability and potentiates the activity of kinins. It, therefore, plays an important role in acute inflammation. PGE_1 is formed from the substrate arachidonic acid and the inhibition of its activity by aspirin and indomethacin is considered to be the basis of the anti-inflammatory activity of these compounds.

2.11 Phagocytosis is promoted by:
1. hyaluronidase
2. neuraminidase
3. the hexose monophosphate shunt
4. immunoglobulin
5. complement

1. False
Hyaluronidase plays no part in phagocytosis. It is, however, an important factor in the spread of infections caused by clostridia, staphylococci and streptococci all of which secrete this enzyme. Its action is to break down hyaluronic acid which is a normal constituent of intercellular ground substance.

2. False
Neuraminidase plays no part in phagocytosis. This substance is an enzyme produced by certain viruses and bacteria which splits a chemical bond between neuraminic acid and other sugars. Neuraminic acid is an important structural component of the surface glycoproteins of many cells.

3. False
The hexose monophosphate shunt does not promote phagocytosis but it is a significant factor in causing the death of microorganisms following phagocytosis. This shunt is a powerful system of enzymes present in polymorphonuclear leucocytes and macrophages. It involves the activation of NADH and NADPH oxidases leading to the formation of powerful oxidising agents including hydrogen peroxide.

4. True
Specific antibodies are important agents in the opsonisation of bacteria prior to phagocytosis.

5. True
Complement components have an action which was known in the past as non-specific opsonisation. The conversion of C3 through either the classical or alternative pathway leads to the formation of C3b. This is recognised by specific cell receptors, by a process of immune adherence, leading to phagocytosis.

2.12 Microorganisms which have undergone phagocytosis are killed by:
1. lecithinase
2. lysozyme

3. lysosomal enzymes
4. lymphokine
5. hydrogen peroxide

1. False
This enzyme has no action on microorganisms. It is one of the many enzymes produced by the clostridia, its specific action is to haemolyse erythrocytes by attacking their cell membranes.

2. True
This enzyme, which is found in the polymorphonuclear leucocytes and at many other sites including tears, plays an important role in the destruction of microorganisms. It acts by destroying the muramic acid-N-acetyl-gluronic bond found in the glycopeptide coat of all bacteria.

3. True
The lysosomal enzymes are a group of proteolytic and hydrolytic enzymes capable of digesting ingested microorganisms. High concentrations of these enzymes are secreted around ingested bacteria following fusion of lysosomes with the phagosome.

4. False
Lymphokines play no direct part in the destruction of ingested micro-organisms. However, these substances do activate the macrophages causing an increased production of lysosomal enzymes. Lymphokines are produced by the action of specific antigens or mitogens on primed T lymphocytes. They are important in the body's defence against certain microorganisms and are concerned with delayed hypersensitivity reactions.

5. True
The killing of bacteria is largely accomplished by oxygen dependent mechanisms. The generation of oxygen metabolites due to the rapid activation of an oxidase (NADPH oxidase) which oxidises NADPH (reduced nicotinamide-adenosine dinucleotide phosphate) and in the process, reduces oxygen to superoxide ion which is then converted to H_2O_2. The concentration of O_2 of itself is insufficient to kill bacteria, but the granules of the neutrophils contain the enzyme myeloperoxidase which in the presence of Cl- converts H_2O to HOCl. This then destroys the organism by binding covalently to bacterial constituents or by oxidation of proteins and lipids.

2.13   Pus contains:
1. lipids
2. fibrin
3. collagen
4. plasma cells
5. polymorphonuclear leucocytes

1. True
Lipids are present in pus. They are derived from the plasma lipoproteins and from cellular breakdown products. Cholesterol may be found in old pus.

2. True
Pus contains fibrin because the activation of the coagulation system by the Hageman factor converts plasma fibrinogen into fibrin. The Hageman factor, Factor XII in the international classification of plasma coagulation factors, may be activated by kallikrein.

3. False
Collagen is not a constituent of pus although its breakdown products may be present due to the activity of enzymes known as collagenases. During healing collagen is laid down by fibroblasts.

4. False
Plasma cells are not normally found in the pus formed as a result of acute inflammation. Chiefly they are found, together with lymphocytes, in the lymph nodes, spleen and gut but they are also present in the organised granulomas which form in 'chronic inflammatory' lesions such as those which develop in rheumatoid arthritis.

5. True
The major cellular component of pus consists of living or dead polymorphonuclear leucocytes. These cells, when living, destroy ingested microorganisms, if these are the cause of the acute inflammatory process. Polymorphonuclear leucocytes are attracted to the site of an acute inflammatory reaction by a variety of chemotactic agents, one of the most potent of which in vitro is a lysate of the polymorphonuclear leucocytes themselves.

2.14 Septicaemia is associated with:
1. bacteraemia
2. toxaemia
3. the multiplication of bacteria in the blood stream
4. invasion of the blood stream by organisms multiplying elsewhere, e.g. the peritoneum
5. multiple haemorrhagic foci in the tissues

1. False
The term bacteraemia implies that bacteria are circulating but not multiplying in the blood stream. Nevertheless, a bacteraemia can be dangerous because any bacteria in the blood stream may settle in various parts of the body. For example, osteomyelitis in children is believed to follow bacteraemia, the responsible organism, commonly the *Staphylococcus aureus*, being deposited in the metaphysis of the long bones.

2. True
Profound toxaemia with high fever complicates a septicaemia because of the toxins liberated from the responsible bacteria. These toxins are pyrogenic of themselves and also cause the formation of pyrogens due to tissue damage.

3. True
The essential feature of a septicaemia is the multiplication of bacteria in the blood stream. An example is infection by the plague bacillus, *Yersinia pestis*.

4. True
In patients suffering from severe peritonitis caused by *Escherichia coli* the organisms in the blood stream are invaders from the inflamed peritoneal cavity.

5. True
Small haemorrhages commonly occur in various organs and tissues. These are caused either by the effects of the accompanying toxaemia on the endothelium or by metastatic foci of bacterial growth.

SECTION 3. CHRONIC INFLAMMATION AND GRANULOMA FORMATION

3.1   Necrosis occurs as a concomitant feature of chronic inflammation in:
1. leprosy
2. tuberculosis
3. syphilis
4. actinomycosis
5. coccidiomycosis

1. False
Necrosis is an inconspicuous feature of both tuberculoid and lepromatous leprosy. In the former epithelioid cell granuloma are the chief feature and leprosy bacilli are often difficult to find. In lepromatous leprosy, the essential lesions are formed of aggregates of mononuclear cells in which large numbers of the lepra bacilli can be found. The so-called 'lepra cells'. The pathogenicity of *Myco. leprae* is so low that the mononuclear cells survive intense parasitism for long periods.

2. True
The characteristic central caseous area of the typical tubercle caused by the *Mycobacterium tuberculosis* is due to necrosis. Caseous material contains a high content of lipid and frequently a large number of bacilli. Aggregation of the follicles finally leads to the development of a tuberculous abscess and if liquefaction of the

caseous material occurs the abscess begins to track through or along tissue planes to form in some cases the typical collar stud or psoas abscess.

3. True
Coagulative necrosis and caseation is typical of the gumma formed in tertiary syphilis. How the necrosis is brought about remains doubtful but it may be due to ischaemia caused by the associated endarteritis obliterans.

4. True
Necrosis is typical of an advanced actinomycotic lesion caused by the *Actinomyces bovis*, a bacterium related to the mycobacteria. The centre of an actinomycotic lesion consists of pus in which is found the 'sulphur granules' which are grey-yellow in colour formed by colonies of filaments resembling fungal mycelia.

5. True
Coccidiomycosis is a fungal infection. The pulmonary lesion is morphologically similar to that of tuberculosis being accompanied by central necrosis and causing micro-abscesses. These lesions frequently become calcified. Healing is associated with the development of a positive coccidioidin delayed hypersensitivity skin reaction.

3.2 The following belong to the mononuclear phagocyte system:
1. macrophages
2. mast cells
3. epithelioid cells
4. fibroblasts
5. Küpffer cells

1. True
The macrophage is the prototype of the cells belonging to the mononuclear phagocyte system. One of the most important characteristics of this cell which was first described by Metchnikoff is its ability to phagocytose foreign particulate and colloidal particles, but they are also important in processing antigen for lymphocyte recognition. It is the active non-specific effector cell in cell-mediated immunity and in host resistance to infection by facultative and obligate intracellular microorganisms, e.g. mycobacteria, protozoa and viruses. Macrophages are derived from bone marrow precursors via circulating monocytes and they are easily recognised histologically by observing their uptake of carbon particles.

2. False
Mast cells are not a part of the MPS. They are the effector cells of IgE induced allergic reactions. Degranulated by antigen-antibody complexes they release histamine and other vasoactive substances such as serotonin and SRS-A.

3. True
Epithelioid cells represent an activated form of the cells of the MPS; they are, however, poorly phagocytic but possess intense enzymatic activity. Such cells are found in the centre of immunologically induced tuberculoid-type granulomas and they may aggregate to form the Langhans type of giant cell.

4. False
Fibroblasts are not related to the mononuclear phagocyte system although they may be found in close proximity to macrophages and epithelioid cells in granulomas. The function of fibroblasts is to secrete collagen.

5. True
Küpffer cells are derived from precursor cells in the bone marrow that circulate as monocytes and then settle in the sinuses of the liver forming actively phagocytic cells.

3.3   Malignant disease may complicate the following chronic inflammatory diseases:
1. chronic osteomyelitis
2. sarcoidosis
3. asbestosis
4. schistosomiasis
5. ulcerative colitis

1. True
Although extremely rare, squamous cell cancers were in the past seen in and around the skin sinuses associated with chronic osteomyelitis. The present rarity of the condition is due to the more effective treatment of osteomyelitis in the acute stage. The incidence of chronic osteomyelitis with the development of a large involucrum and chronically draining sinuses is extremely low in the Western World.

2. False
Sarcoidosis is not associated with malignant change.

3. True
Asbestosis is associated with the development of both squamous cell carcinoma and mesothelioma, 60% of the latter being due to exposure to asbestos, this relationship being first noted in South Africa. The fibre type associated with mesothelioma is crocidolite and the latent interval between exposure and the development of the tumour itself may be as long as 40 years. Such tumours occurring in the lungs are not necessarily associated with pulmonary fibrosis.

4. True
This disease is due to infestation with the dioecious trematodes, *Schistosoma haematobium, mansoni and japonicum*. In Egypt the predominant infection is with *S. haematobium* and the adult parasites

lie in the veins of the bladder. The eggs laid by the female pass into the submucosa and excite a granulomatous reaction which is later followed by metaplasia of the transitional cell urothelium to a squamous type. Squamous cell carcinoma then develops in a proportion of the victims, particularly infected Egyptians.

5. True
It is now well recognised that ulcerative colitis is a 'premalignant condition'. The incidence of malignancy increasing with the duration and totality of the disease being rarely seen in its more distal forms. At least one third of all cases with a history longer than 12 years develop cancer, usually multifocally.

3.4 **Accumulation of macrophages is a prominent histological feature of the lesions produced by the following diseases:**
1. leishmaniasis
2. extrinsic allergic alveolitis
3. Gaucher's disease
4. legionnaire's disease
5. Letterer–Siwe's disease

1. True
Both cutaneous leishmaniasis (oriental sore) and systemic leishmaniasis (kala-azar) are associated with lesions in which a particular feature is the large number of macrophages present. These contain the Leishman–Donovan bodies which are the amastigote form of the parasite.

2. False
One example of extrinsic allergic alveolitis is farmer's lung which is caused by the inhalation of the spores of *Micropolyspora faeni* found in mouldy hay. The lesion is caused by the deposition of immune complexes which activate complement giving rise to pulmonary fibrosis.

3. True
Gaucher's disease, an inherited condition, is due to a defect in the enzyme β-glucocerebrosidase. As a result large quantities of glucocerebroside accumulates in the macrophages especially of the spleen and to a lesser extent in the liver and lymph nodes of the thorax and abdomen. Such cells known as the Gaucher cells are large, up to 80 μm in diameter, with a pale cytoplasm in which is an irregular network of fibrils.

4. False
A severe form of pyogenic bronchopneumonia with an almost lobar distribution, the disease occurs in epidemics and is believed to be caused by a Gram-negative bacillus, *Legionella*. The organism requires special cultures and tissue sections require staining with silver in order to demonstrate the pathogen.

5. True
A form of 'histiocytosis X' which is a term applied to three conditions, Letterer–Siwe's disease, Hand–Schüller–Christian disease and eosinophil granuloma of bone. The condition referred to occurs in infancy and early childhood and runs a rapidly fatal course. It is characterized by hepatosplenomegaly, lymphadenopathy and multiple nodules in the skin and bone marrow. The affected organs show massive replacement by proliferated macrophage-like cells which are swollen, pale and contain phagocytosed debris.

3.5   Hyperplasia of the lymphoid tissue is a prominent feature in the following conditions:
1. toxoplasmosis
2. leishmaniasis
3. chronic dermatitis
4. silicosis
5. berylliosis

1. True
Lymph node enlargement, caused chiefly by a reactive hyperplasia of all components of the node, is a prominent feature of toxoplasmosis, caused by infection with the protozoan, *Toxoplasma gondii*. In addition the germinal centres are larger than those observed in similar infections and contain scattered accumulations of epithelioid type macrophages and B lymphocytes. The infection occurs in man due to accidentally ingesting oocytes from cat faeces or from eating incompletely cooked lamb or pork. Infection with this protozoan is especially serious in the foetus or in immunocompromised individuals.

2. False
Specific hyperplasia of the lymphoid tissues does not occur in cutaneous leishmaniasis, otherwise known as oriental sore, caused by the protozoan, *Leishmania tropica*. In the systemic form of the disease, kala-azar caused by *Leishmania donovani*, hepatosplenomegaly occurs due to collections of macrophages which contain the Leishman–Donovan bodies. The latter are parasitic amastigotes.

3. True
Chronic dermatitis is associated with dermatopathic lymphadenopathy in which there may be replacement of paracortical areas with macrophages and enlargement of the germinal centres.

4. False
Silicosis does not appear to affect lymphoid tissue except to cause fibrosis. Fibrosis of inguinal lymphoid tissue is thought to be a cause of non-filarial elephantiasis in Ethiopia, as a result of absorption of silica through the skin.

5. False
Beryllium oxide dust, when inhaled, produces progressive pulmonary fibrosis with associated loss of pulmonary function. The precise

mechanism by which the pathological changes occur remains unknown, although a Type IV hypersensitivity reaction may play a part in the pathological process.

3.6   Giant cells are characteristically found in the pathological lesions associated with the following diseases:
1. actinomycosis
2. schistosomiasis
3. primary biliary cirrhosis
4. lepromatous leprosy
5. Hodgkin's disease

1. False
Actinomycosis is caused by a 'higher bacterium', the *A. israeli*. Infection with this organism produces chronic granulomatous abscesses most commonly in the facio-maxillary region. The abscess wall is heavily infiltrated with lipid laden macrophages and within the abscess are found mycelial masses between 0.2–2 mm in diameter, the 'sulphur granules', on the periphery of which are club-shaped swellings which are believed to be deposited by the host's tissue cells as a reaction to the presence of the organism.

2. False
The granulomas associated with schistosomiasis form around the eggs which are laid by the female in the veins of the walls of the lower urinary tract in the case of *S. haematobium*. Occasional epithelioid cells, fibroblasts, lymphocytes and plasma cells are seen but giant cells are not a special feature.

3. True
Primary biliary cirrhosis, a disease affecting middle-aged women rather than men, is of unknown aetiology. Pathologically a non-suppurative process affects the intrahepatic bile ducts. Miliary granuloma form in the portal areas associated with a heavy infiltration of lymphoid cells and some giant cells.

4. False
In contradistinction to tuberculoid leprosy in which the lesions resemble those of tuberculosis, giant cells are rarely found in the lepromatous variety of this disease. In lepromatous leprosy the lesions consist of aggregates of macrophages which contain huge numbers of lepra bacilli. The bacilli tend not to be destroyed and to multiply within the cells which have ingested them.

5. True
The characteristic cell of Hodgkin's disease is the Sternberg–Reed giant cell. This cell possesses double mirror image nuclei and is a particular feature of the pleomorphic cellular infiltrate which replaces the normal lymphoid tissue. The cells are probably neoplastic cells derived from the mononuclear phagocyte system.

3.7   The following predispose to the development of tuberculosis:
1. HLA–B27
2. sarcoidosis
3. silicosis
4. avitaminosis D
5. malnutrition

1. False
The histocompatibility antigen HLA–B27 is not associated with an increased predisposition to tuberculosis but is associated with a high incidence of ankylosing spondylitis and acute anterior uveitis.

2. False
Tuberculosis is rarely associated with sarcoidosis and the tuberculin reaction is frequently negative. However, the pathological lesion in the lungs and lymph nodes resembles that of a tuberculoid granuloma but without any associated caseation.

3. True
There appears to be a synergism between silicosis and tuberculosis and in the presence of the former the incidence of the latter is greatly increased. Once the mycobacterium becomes established the disease may rapidly progress terminating in tuberculous bronchopneumonia and miliary tuberculosis.

4. False
Although vitamin D was used in the treatment of tuberculosis and particularly for lupus vulgaris, there is no evidence that a deficiency of this vitamin predisposes to the development of tuberculosis any more than a general state of malnutrition.

5. True
Protein-calorie malnutrition results in low resistance to a wide range of infections. Children with kwashiorkor have a depressed tuberculin reactivity and a lowered resistance to infection with mycobacteria.

3.8   Direct evidence of immunological activity can be demonstrated in the following chronic inflammatory diseases:
1. lepromatous leprosy
2. tuberculoid leprosy
3. silicosis
4. rheumatoid arthritis
5. asbestosis   .

1. False
Granuloma associated with lepromatous leprosy consist of diffuse collections of macrophages, within which are large numbers of *Myco. leprae* cells in which the bacteria have undergone degeneration and become distended with a lipid substance derived from the capsule of the bacilli. These large fat-distended cells or globi retain eosinophilic

fragments of the organism at their periphery and are a diagnostic feature. No significant infiltration of lymphocytes or plasma cells occurs around these lesions and the lepromin test is negative.

2. True
Tuberculoid leprosy causes a non-caseating epithelioid cell granuloma in which the typical lesion is surrounded by a dense cuff of lymphocytes, together with epithelioid cells which often form Langhans giant cells. The lepromin test is positive and evidence of T-lymphocyte activation can be found in vitro.

3. False
Patients suffering from silicosis may develop autoantibodies but these are not directly involved in the pathogenesis of the silicotic nodules which are formed from collagen. Colloidal silica is intensely toxic to macrophages and it is this damage, with the release of intracellular lysosomes, which appears to stimulate the intense fibroblastic activity.

4. True
The microscopic appearance of the early lesions of rheumatoid arthritis is evidence of the immunological aetiology of this disease. Such lesions consist of a central area of necrosis and fibroblastic activity surrounded by a cuff of lymphocytes and plasma cells. The latter appear to produce the rheumatoid factor which is an IgM anti-immunoglobulin antibody.

5. False
No evidence of immunological activity is seen in the lesions produced by asbestos, another silica containing material which in fibre form can react with the macrophage cell membrane to cause intense fibroblastic activity and collagen synthesis. When inhaled this reactive lesion is found particularly around the terminal bronchioles as well as the air sacs.

3.9 Epithelioid cell granuloma formation is associated with the following diseases:
1. ulcerative colitis
2. Crohn's disease
3. chronic glomerulo-nephritis
4. toxoplasmosis
5. sarcoidosis

1. False
This condition, which is a chronic inflammatory disease of the colon, is not associated with granuloma formation. Characteristically the disease, in its later and more severe forms, is associated with mucosal denudation due to the coalescence of smaller ulcers which develop from crypt abscesses. Such ulceration seldom extends more deeply than the submucosa.

2. True
In the early acute phase of this disease a non-specific infiltration of chronic inflammatory cells consisting of plasma cells, macrophages and eosinophil cells is present. In the later granulomatous stage epithelioid and multinuclear giant cells appear in 'sarcoid like' non-caseating follicles. The inflammatory process may extend through the whole thickness of the affected viscus, thus involving the peritoneal surface of the abdominal viscera; hence the development of internal fistulas. In the later stages fibrosis becomes increasingly prominent resulting in the development of strictures.

3. False
Organised granulomas do not occur in this condition although fibrosis around the glomerular tufts leads to their deformation. This disease is attributed to chronic immune complex deposition.

4. True
Small epithelioid cell granulomas may be a feature of the lesions of toxoplasmosis, a disease caused by the protozoan, *Toxoplasma gondii*. They may be found in the enlarged lymph nodes which typically occur in this infection.

5. True
Sarcoidosis is a disease of unknown aetiology in which lesions found in the lungs and lymph nodes are typically non-caseating tuberculoid granulomas. These may be followed by intense pulmonary fibrosis. The diagnosis can be made by the use of the Kveim test in which an extract of the spleen of an affected individual is injected intradermally into the patient under investigation. A positive test results in the development of an organised epithelioid cell granuloma within six weeks.

3.10 Organised epithelioid cell granulomas develop in the following infections:
1. leprosy
2. syphilis
3. ankylostomiasis
4. ascariasis
5. schistosomiasis

1. True
Epithelioid granulomas develop in the tuberculoid and not in the lepromatous form of leprosy. In the former the granulomas are immunologically induced and the positive Mitsuda type of skin reaction which develops within 2 to 3 weeks of the intradermal injection of dead *Mycobacterium leprae* is also an epithelioid cell granuloma. In contrast the granulomas associated with lepromatous leprosy are not immunologically induced, contain no epithelioid cells and the Mitsuda test is negative.

2. True

Gummas are nodular masses of syphylitic granulation tissue varying in size from scarcely visible lesions to masses several cm in size. The centre of the lesion undergoes necrosis and the periphery of the lesion is surrounded by an extensive zone of lymphocytes and plasma cells. Epithelioid cells may be found in follicles together with giant cells, the latter being smaller than the Langhans cells found in tuberculosis. Since the necrotic centre does not undergo softening, a gumma remains firm and rubbery.

3. False

Hookworm infection is not associated with granuloma formation. Transient pulmonary eosinophilia occurs in this condition if the larvae penetrate the intestinal wall and migrate through the lungs. Individuals suffering from ankylostomiasis usually have a severe anaemia due to the induced gastrointestinal haemorrhage.

4. False

Infection with the round worm, *Ascaris lumbricoides*, which is particularly prevalent in tropical areas, is not associated with granulomatous formation. Severe infection with round worms causes malnutrition and by entwining themselves into a bolus may cause intestinal obstruction or migrating into the common bile duct, cholangitis. The eggs hatch in the small intestine and having penetrated the gut wall are carried in the circulation to the lungs. Bursting through the alveolar capillaries, they travel upwards to the pharynx and are swallowed to develop into adult worms in the small intestine. Migration of the larvae to the lungs causes pulmonary eosinophilia. Eosinophilia and a high IgE level are common in infected individuals.

5. True

The granulomas developing around schistosome eggs in the liver, intestines and bladder are typical immunologically induced epithelioid cell granulomas, usually associated with lymphocytes, plasma cells and eosinophils. Large numbers of fibroblasts are present and so these lesions are followed by intense fibrosis.

3.11 The following metals cause epithelioid cell granulomas:
  1. beryllium
  2. chromium
  3. zirconium
  4. nickel
  5. iron

1. True

The inhalation of beryllium is followed by a chronic inflammatory response in the lung. Commonly a non-caseating tuberculoid reaction is seen in the tissues. In addition to this action beryllium is a contact sensitising metal.

2. False
Potassium dichromate does not cause granuloma formation but it does cause severe contact sensitivity. This particularly affects workers in the building trade because it may be a constituent of cement. Chromium used in orthopaedic implants can also cause sensitisation leading to local tissue breakdown and generalized skin rashes.

3. True
The metal itself is inert. However, zirconium lactate can cause non-caseating tuberculoid granulomas in the skin, the development of which are due to delayed hypersensitivity.

4. False
Nickel does not cause granulomas but like potassium dichromate it is a contact sensitiser. It may also give rise to local tissue reactions if used in orthopaedic implants.

5. False
No tissue reaction occurs in response to iron or its various salts. However, in persons who have inhaled iron compounds over long periods an X-ray of the lungs gives a false impression that multiple granulomas have developed. No evidence of a chronic inflammatory lesion is, however, found in lung biopsies performed in such individuals.

SECTION 4. HOSPITAL AND WOUND INFECTION

4.1   Infection within a hospital may be:
1. dust-borne
2. water-borne
3. food-borne
4. hand-borne
5. endogenous

1. True
Infected particles redistributed from a static position by dusting or bed making may lead to respiratory tract infections. A further possibility is the distribution of such particles through inadequate or imperfectly maintained ventilation systems. Droplet nuclei 1–10 μm in diameter formed by the evaporation of small droplets may remain in the air for long periods and are accountable for some virus infections such as the common cold.

2. True
Water-borne infection may occur due to contamination of a water supply with excreta. This is the common method of spread of cholera and typhoid fever.

3. True

Food-borne infection is usually the result of infection of the food supplied to patients by foodhandlers who are carrying an intestinal pathogen. Alternatively if infected water is used for washing food infection may be transmitted.

4. True

Hand-borne infections are usually due to poor personal hygiene. Patients and carriers with intestinal pathogens can contaminate their hands with traces of faeces when cleansing themselves after defaecation.

5. True

Endogenous infection is common particularly in patients in whom the original disease was the result of bacterial infection, e.g. peritonitis following appendicitis or diverticulitis.

4.2   General factors predisposing to wound infection include:
1. uncontrolled diabetes
2. hypogammaglobulinaemia
3. low platelet count
4. agranulocytopenia
5. eosinophilia

1. True

The defective carbohydrate metabolism of diabetes results in a diminished supply of energy for the polymorphonuclear leucocytes, thus diminishing their phagocytic potential.

2. True

Because all antibodies are gammaglobulins it follows that hypogammaglobulinaemia is associated with a failure of antibody formation and hence a reduction of one of the important factors concerned in resistance to infection.

3. True

This statement is true only because severe thrombocytopenia predisposes to the development of a wound haematoma, a common precursor of wound infection.

4. True

In agranulocytosis the polymorphonuclear leucocytes suddenly disappear from the blood. Since these cells are a major factor in the defence against pathogenic microorganisms, agranulocytosis leads to a greatly increased susceptibility to infection which may be rapidly fatal. In about one third of all cases no cause can be found and in the remainder the chief causes include a number of drugs including phenybutazone, PAS, phenothiazines and thiouracil.

5. False

Although the eosinophil leucocyte does migrate into inflamed areas they play little part in the body's defences against bacterial infection.

They are more conspicuous in hypersensitivity reactions and infestation with various kinds of worms.

4.3   The following diseases are the result of arthropod-borne blood infections:
1. cholera
2. trypanosomiasis
3. tetanus
4. malaria
5. hydatid disease

1. False
Cholera is a water-borne infection, transmission taking place by the faecal-oral route.

2. True
Trypanosomiasis is transmitted by the tsetse fly. *T. gambiense* is transmitted mainly by intra-human cycles whereas *T. rhodesiense* is a zoonosis.

3. False
Tetanus is due to the Gram-positive *Clostridium tetani* which is found in the soil often in spore form. Following injury the spore contaminates the wound and develops into the vegetative toxin producing form only if conditions are anaerobic.

4. True
Malaria is transmitted by the anopheles mosquito. The disease is caused by one of four species of plasmodium: *Plasmodium vivax, malariae, ovale* or *falciparum.* The latter is the most important.

5. False
Hydatid disease is caused by the tapeworms, *Echinococcus granulosus* and *multilocularis.* The natural cycle is from dog to sheep and man is infected only by accident.

4.4   *Streptococcus faecalis:*
1. is a common inhabitant of the gastrointestinal tract
2. grows in long chains
3. flourishes in bile-salt lactose media
4. is concerned in the aetiology of periodontal disease
5. is an opportunistic rather than a true pathogen

1. True
Streptococcus faecalis is almost as numerous in the faeces of man as the bacteroides, bifidobacteria and enterobacteriaceae.

2. False
This organism occurs in pairs looking like spectacles or at the most, in short chains.

3. True
Streptococcus faecalis grows on MacConkey's medium and other bile-salt lactose media to produce very small pink colonies. Normally no change occurs on a blood agar plate although a variant exists which causes a clear zone of haemolysis without producing a soluble haemolysin.

4. True
The superficial dental plaques which form in the angle around the crown of the tooth just above the margin of the gum are inhabited by *Streptococcus mutans, mitis* and *faecalis*. When the mouth is not kept clean this marginal plaque grows down into the gingival crevice and induces a change in the bacterial flora to one dominated by anaerobic Gram-negative cocci, bacilli, vibrios and spirochaetes. The toxins and enzymes produced by these various organisms accompanied by the immune response to their antigens damages the periodontal tissues causing the development of gingivitis and pyorrhoea.

5. True
Streptococcus faecalis is an opportunistic pathogen. Unlike a true pathogen it can only produce a pathological lesion in the presence of a lowered tissue resistance or abnormal environmental conditions.

4.5 The virulence of bacteria is related to:
1. their number in the tissues
2. the production of toxins
3. their ability to produce spreading factors
4. their resistance to phagocytosis
5. decreased resistance of the host

1. False
The number of bacteria does not affect their virulence, only their potential for producing an infective lesion. About 10^5 coagulase positive staphylococci are required to produce a superficial infective lesion such as a boil.

2. True
Bacterial toxins are of two main types, exotoxins and endotoxins. Both play a large part in determining bacterial virulence. The former, which are mainly produced by Gram-positive organisms, diffuse freely from the organisms into the surrounding tissues although some, like the exotoxin of *Clostridium tetani* have an affinity for specific tissues. Endotoxins, however, are an integral part of the cell. Typical examples are the glyco-lipid complexes of the Gram-negative organisms such as *Escherichia coli*.

3. True
Spreading factors, such as streptokinase which is produced by *Streptococcus pyogenes*, are important factors in determining bacterial virulence. This enzyme activates a proteolytic enzyme

precursor in the plasma and causes the lysis of fibrin clots. Another factor of similar importance is hyaluronidase which is produced by *Clostridium perfringens* and other organisms. This enzyme splits hyaluronic acid, the muco-polysaccharide intercellular cement substance, thus enabling the clostridia to spread along the tissue planes.

4. True
Resistance to phagocytosis chiefly depends upon the presence of surface components on the bacteria which make it difficult for the phagocytic cells to ingest them. Virulent strains of pneumococci, for example, possess polysaccharide capsules, whereas rough mutants which have lost their capsules are readily engulfed by phagocytes.

5. False
Decreased resistance of the host does not affect the inherent virulence of the organism. It does, however, affect the number required to produce a clinical lesion. In an experimental animal the minimum lethal dose of organisms would also be reduced.

4.6   Bacteria are normally found on or in the:
1. blood
2. urinary tract
3. lower bronchi
4. gastrointestinal tract
5. skin, sebaceous glands and hair follicles

1. False
In a normal individual bacteria are only transiently found in the blood stream, e.g. following tooth brushing. Such bacteria do not multiply and are rapidly eliminated.

2. False
The urinary tract is normally sterile. Infection of the female urethra with Gram-negative cocci, however, is the common cause of the urethral syndrome, often mistakenly referred to as 'cystitis' although the bladder urine is sterile.

3. False
The lower bronchi are normally sterile.

4. True
The gastrointestinal tract is inhabited by an abundant bacterial flora from the level of the duodenojejunal junction onwards. It has only recently been appreciated, however, that obligate anaerobes belonging to the bacteroides group constitute a majority of the intestinal flora. Prior to culture of the small bowel contents using anaerobic techniques, it was thought that this part of the bowel was sterile.

5. True
Staphylococcus albus, Staphylococcus aureus, diphtheroid

organisms, lactobacilli and a variety of obligate anaerobes colonise the skin and its appendages.

4.7   Pseudomembranous enterocolitis is caused by the following organisms:
1. *Clostridium sporogenes*
2. *Clostridium difficile*
3. *Streptococcus faecalis*
4. penicillin resistant staphylococci
5. *Pseudomonas aeruginosa*

1. False
Clostridium sporogenes is one of the causative organisms of gas gangrene, it plays no part in the development of enterocolitis.

2. True
Clostridium difficile has recently been identified as the causal agent of antibiotic associated colitis. The organism is resistant to both lincomycin and clindamycin and exerts its noxious effect through the production of cytopathic toxin. The organism is sensitive to vancomycin and metranidazole.

3. False
Streptococcus faecalis plays no part in the development of pseudomembranous enterocolitis. This organism is an opportunistic pathogen and can only produce a pathological lesion when tissue resistance is lowered.

4. True
Penicillin resistant staphylococci are believed to play a part in the development of one type of pseudomembranous enterocolitis. This type of enterocolitis was particularly common in the past, when broad spectrum antibiotics were used over prolonged periods in an attempt to reduce post-operative wound infection.

5. False
Pseudomonas aeruginosa plays no part in the development of pseudomembranous enterocolitis. This organism is of considerable importance, however, in burns when the burnt surface tends to be colonised by this organism producing the characteristic greenish pus.

4.8   The major pathogens in post operative chest infections are:
1. *Haemophilus influenzae*
2. *Streptococcus pyogenes*
3. *Mycobacterium tuberculosis*
4. *Staphylococcus aureus*
5. *Streptococcus pneumoniae*

1. True
This organism is one of the most important pathogens concerned in the development of post operative chest infections particularly in

patients in whom pulmonary collapse occurs. This organism is sensitive to the cephalosporin group of antibiotics.

2. False
This organism plays no part in the development of post operative pulmonary infection. It is, however, an important pathogen causing acute tonsillitis, impetigo, wound infections, otitis media, scarlet and rheumatic fever.

3. False
Mycobacterium tuberculosis, although a cause of severe chronic pulmonary infection, plays no part in the development of post operative chest infection.

4. True
Staphylococcus aureus may be of importance in post operative chest infections but only in the presence of a staphylococcal septicaemia. Typically it causes multiple small abscesses to develop within the lungs.

5. True
Streptococcus pneumoniae is the chief pathogenic invader of the lungs, normally producing lobar pneumonia. Since post operative pulmonary infection is normally limited to areas involved in collapse the classical picture does not develop. It should also be noted that the majority of pathogenic bacteria, chlamydia, rickettsia, viruses and fungi are potential causes of post operative chest infection although all are uncommon.

4.9   The following bacteria are commonly found in infected wounds following colonic operations:
1. *Escherichia coli*
2. *Neisseria meningitidis*
3. *Streptococcus pyogenes*
4. *Streptococcus faecalis*
5. *Bacteroides fragilis*

1. True
Escherichia coli belongs to a group of bacteria known as the *Enterobacteriaceae*, many members of which are responsible for wound infections. Other than *E. coli* these include *Klebsiella aerogenes* and *Proteus mirabilis*.

2. False
Neisseria meningitidis is a coccal organism, normally a commensal in the nasopharynx which plays no part in wound infection but is, of course, the causal organism of acute meningococcal meningitis.

3. True
A microaerophilic streptococcus may be involved in wound infection following colonic operations. If combined with other organisms such as *Proteus mirabilis* or *Staphylococcus aureus* a progressive

synergistic gangrene may develop often referred to as Melaney's synergistic gangrene. This type of gangrene is particularly common in obese patients, black necrotic sloughs developing on the abdominal wall.

4. True
Streptococcus faecalis is a commensal of the large intestine and may be involved in any wound infection following colonic surgery.

5. True
The part played by *Bacteroides fragilis* has only recently been appreciated since it was common clinical practice to culture all wound swabs taken from infected wounds under aerobic conditions. Since *Bact. fragilis* is a strict anaerobe its presence in wound infections was, therefore, unrecognised.

4.10 The incidence of postoperative infection can be reduced by the use of the following measures:
1. the use of negative pressure ventilation in the operating theatre
2. the use of filtered air in the operating theatre, pore size 10 μm
3. showering by the surgeon and all attendants prior to embarking upon the operation
4. the administration of prophylactic antibiotics
5. disinfection of the patient's skin prior to operation

1. False
The most commonly used system of theatre ventilation is a positive pressure (plenum) system. Although there are various methods by which this can be achieved the downward displacement method is the most popular. In this type of system filtered air is introduced into the theatre from ports in the ceiling and air is extracted from floor level.

2. False
This is too large. The most commonly used filters have pores of approximately 5 μm in diameter. Pores smaller than this are unnecessary since the organisms are never solitary but are usually to be found on dust particles. One problem encountered with a smaller pore size is the difficulty of maintaining the filters which rapidly become blocked.

3. False
Showering is not a practice which is to be recommended since it removes the oil from the surface skin to which organisms normally adhere. The result is that any movement by the surgeon or attendants will be attended by a shower of organisms.

4. True
Prophylactic antibiotics have been shown to be effective in reducing the incidence of post operative wound infection in a variety of potentially infective conditions such as acute appendicitis, acute

cholecystitis and colonic operations. At the present time clindamycin or metranidazole are being used with increasing frequency.

5. True
Disinfection of the patient's skin prior to surgery is regarded as an essential prerequisite of aseptic surgery. This may be carried out by a variety of materials. At present the iodophors or chlorhexidine are commonly used for this purpose.

4.11 Renal tract infection is caused by a variety of bacteria including:
1. *Streptococcus pyogenes*
2. *Klebsiella pneumoniae*
3. *Streptococcus faecalis*
4. *Staphylococcus aureus*
5. *Escherichia coli*

1. False
This organism is associated with the development of progressive glomerulonephritis. In this latter situation fluorescent microscopy reveals a granular deposition of IgG and complement in the walls of the glomerular capillaries.

2. True
Otherwise known as *Freidlander's bacillus* this organism is most commonly found in mixed infections and in the presence of structural deformities of the urinary tract.

3. True
This organism is a particularly common offender in women, in whom it may be introduced into the renal tract by catheterization causing both cystitis and pyelonephritis.

4. True
Both *Staphylococcus albus* (Coag–ve) and *Staphylococcus aureus* (Coag+ve) can cause pyelonephritis, the former more commonly than the latter. The Coagulase +ve organism is only occasionally found in structurally abnormal urinary tracts.

5. True
This organism is the commonest cause of acute and chronic urinary tract infection.

4.12 Staphylococci pathogenic to man:
1. produce a capsular polysaccharide
2. grow in irregular clusters in culture
3. produce coagulase
4. are resistant to penicillin
5. all produce an enterotoxin

1. False
Capsular polysaccharide is associated with the pathogenic forms of

pneumococci. The presence of a capsule produces the smooth variant, loss of the capsule an avirulent rough form.

2. True
The growth of the staphylococci is irregular thus producing irregular clusters.

3. True
The ability to produce coagulase, an enzyme which clots citrated plasma in vitro, differentiates the pathogenic forms of staphylococci from the nonpathogenic.

4. False
Pathogenic staphylococci are not necessarily resistant to penicillin although most strains associated with epidemic and endemic disease in hospitals in fact are resistant. Resistance to this, or any other antibiotics, affects the treatment of an infection but not the initial pathogenicity of the organisms.

5. False
Only some strains of staphylococci produce an enterotoxin. Food containing such organisms acts as a culture medium and when ingested the toxin gives rise to giddiness, vomiting and diarrhoea. This is often severe but recovery usually occurs within a day or two.

4.13 The common pathogenic pyogenic organisms affecting man include:
1. *Staphylococcus aureus*
2. *Clostridium tetani*
3. *Staphylococcus albus*
4. bacteroides
5. *Pseudomonas aeruginosa*

1. True
The pathogenic varieties of this Gram-positive organism are particularly associated with:
    (a) The development of localized infections such as boils, carbuncles and abscesses
    (b) Spreading infections of the skin such as impetigo
    (c) Septicaemia followed by the formation of pyogenic abscesses, osteomyelitis or endocarditis

2. False
Clostridium tetani is not a pyogenic organism. It causes its pathogenic effects by an exotoxin which diffuses up the peripheral or cranial motor nerves to reach the spinal cord or brain where it interferes with the normal inhibitory control of the lower motor neurons by the higher centres.

3. False
Staphylococcus albus is a commensal and rarely pathogenic; it is extremely common on the skin.

4. True
Bacteroides which are nonsporing anaerobic organisms are the commonest organisms present in the intestines. They are frequently associated in pyogenic infections with other organisms such as the anaerobic cocci. They are a particularly important cause of pus formation in surgical wounds following colo-rectal surgery and with intra-abdominal septic complications. Sometimes carried in the blood, they may cause brain abscesses and septicaemia.

5. True
Normally present in small numbers in the gastrointestinal tract these organisms can cause severe infections in burn patients. The pus produced possesses a characteristic greenish colour. These organisms are also responsible for some urinary tract infections and may invade the blood stream to produce a septicaemia.

SECTION 5. DISINFECTION, STERILIZATION AND ANTIBIOTICS

5.1 When using an autoclave to sterilize surgical drapes and instruments it is essential that:
1. the load should be tightly packed
2. the containers in which the loads are packed should be impervious to steam
3. air should be completely removed from the chamber prior to the admission of steam
4. a vacuum must be made at the end of the cycle
5. an adequate indication of autoclave efficiency should be included in the load

1. False
The loads should not be tightly packed because tight packing hinders the passage of steam into and through the loads thus interfering with sterilization.

2. False
Until recently materials to be sterilized were packed in metal drums and if these remain in use the vents to allow the admission of steam must be opened before placing the drums in the sterilizer. The more modern technique is to wrap materials in paper or Steriseal and place the packs in cages or racks.

3. True
This is a prerequisite for the correct functioning of the modern autoclave which does not depend on gravity displacement. By removing 98% of the air from the chamber penetration of the load occurs almost instantly so that efficient sterilization is obtained and the cycle time is shortened. Normal sterilizing time is 3 minutes at 134°C.

4. True

The creation of a vacuum at the end of the cycle in a chamber still warm from the presence of steam, in both the chamber and the surrounding jacket, ensures that the contents of the autoclave are dry before removal.

5. True

In most departments the Bowie Dick test has been replaced by Lantor Testing daily. This test is performed prior to the day's work in the sterilizing unit, after which the efficacy of the procedure is judged by an automatic recording device which indicates the temperatures reached and the duration of the cycle.

5.2   Spores are killed by exposure to:
1. moist heat at 110°C for 15 minutes
2. dry heat at 160°C for 1 hour
3. ethylene oxide
4. hydrogen peroxide
5. gentian violet

1. False

Bacterial spores require exposure to moist heat at a temperature of 121°C for at least 15 minutes and preferably 30 minutes before they are destroyed. Resistant spores such as the spores of *Clostridium botulinum* can resist autoclaving at the lower temperature of 115°C for up to 40 minutes.

2. True

The majority of spores are killed by exposure to dry heat at 160°C for 1 hour. In practice this is an unacceptable method of sterilization because slight charring of paper and cotton occurs at this temperature.

3. True

Ethylene oxide is highly lethal to all kinds of microbes and spores. It is of particular value for sterilizing articles liable to damage by heat, e.g. plastic and rubber articles. Sterilization time depends upon the temperature of the reaction and the relative humidity.

4. False

Hydrogen peroxide has been used as an antiseptic but has little or no action on bacterial spores.

5. False

Gentian violet will kill some vegetative forms of bacteria particularly Gram-positive organisms. It is much less active against Gram-negative bacteria and virtually useless against spores of any kind.

5.3   Differences between disinfectants and antiseptics are:
1. the latter are more harmful to living tissue cells

2. antiseptics free inanimate objects from vegetative organisms whereas disinfectants are used for the local removal of pathogenic bacteria from the tissues
3. the former are more readily inactivated by contact with proteinaceous material such as blood
4. the speed of action of disinfectants can be accelerated by raising the temperature whereas the action of antiseptics can only be intensified by increasing their concentration.
5. there are specific differences in the mode of action of both groups of compounds

1. False
The converse is correct.

2. False
The converse is correct. Disinfectants are used to free inanimate objects from vegetative organisms but not necessarily from spores whereas antiseptics are primarily bacteriostatic agents for the removal of pathogenic bacteria from the tissues.

3. False
Both are equally affected by proteinaceous material.

4. False
The speed of action of both groups of substances can be accelerated by raising the temperature and/or their concentration.

5. False
Both groups of agents may have a variety of actions including disruption of the cytoplasmic membranes, enzyme systems or cellular proteins.

5.4   Chemical agents used as disinfectants and antiseptics include the following compounds:
1. the phenols
2. isopropyl alcohol
3. the halogens
4. the soaps
5. derivatives of salicylic acid

1. True
Phenol, which is carbolic acid, was used by Lister over 100 years ago, to prevent wound infection. This group of chemical compounds act by coagulating protein. Phenol is effective against both bacteria and viruses but it is no longer used because of its toxicity. However, a variety of derivatives such as lysol, Dettol and hexachlorophine are in common use.

2. True
This compound is in common use for sterilization of the skin and is most effective in 70% concentration. The alcohols act by coagulating cell proteins, thus killing bacteria and some viruses.

3. True

The halogens, or any substance capable of releasing them, such as sodium hypochlorite, are lethal to bacteria, viruses, fungi and spores. Their action is to oxidise SH groups but a disadvantage is their susceptibility to quenching by organic matter.

4. True

Soaps have weak disinfectant activity although they are active against *Strep. pyogenes, Strep. pneumoniae, Haemophilus influenzae* and the virus of influenza. They have no action on *Staph. pyogenes*, mycobacteria or Gram-negative bacilli. The main effect of soap is a mechanical one removing the transient skin flora.

5. False

Salicylic acid and the salicylates have no disinfectant or antiseptic action.

5.5 The following antibiotics are effective against fungi:
1. nystatin
2. bacitracin
3. griseofulvin
4. polymyxin B
5. amphotericin B

1. True

Candida albicans, Cryptococcus neoformans and *Histoplasma capsulatum* and *dubosii* are sensitive to this drug. However, the drug is not absorbed and, therefore, has no systemic effect. Its chief clinical use is, therefore, limited to oropharyngeal, vaginal and skin infections caused by *Candida albicans*.

2. False

Bacitracin is a polypeptide antibiotic which is active against many Gram-positive bacteria and neisseria. It is now only used locally for skin infections.

3. True

This drug is produced by the growth of certain strains of penicillin griseofulvum. It exerts an inhibiting effect on the growth of the epidermophyton causing athlete's foot, the trichophyton causing ring worm and the microsporum causing tinea. Administered orally griseofulvin is partially absorbed and is incorporated into the keratin of skin, nails and hair.

4. False

The polymyxins are polypeptides which are derived from the soil organisms *B. polymyxa*. Five have been identified of which two are in commercial use, polymyxin B (polymyxin) and polymyxin E (coliston). These drugs are effective against both Gram-positive and -negative organisms, particularly *Pseudomonas aeruginosa* but they are inactive against proteus. They have no antifungal action.

5. True
This drug is the most effective agent for the treatment of systemic fungal infections. It is active against *Histoplasma capsulatum* and *dubosii*, *Cryptococcus neoformans*, *Coccidioides immitis*, *Blastomyces dermatitidis* and *Candida albicans*.

5.6   Benzyl penicillin is:
1. bacteriostatic
2. destroyed by the enzyme penicillinase
3. insoluble in water
4. damaging to the nucleus of the bacterial cell
5. active against some viruses

1. False
Benzyl penicillin is bactericidal. In vitro bacteria which have been exposed to this antibiotic die even when transferred to a drug-free medium. Compare this with bacteriostatic drugs such as the tetracyclines. Exposure to a bacteriostatic antibiotic causes the cessation of bacterial growth but division recommences if the organisms are transferred to an antibiotic free medium.

2. True
Penicillinase destroys penicillin by hydrolysis to inactive penicilloic acid and by opening the β-lactam ring.

3. False
Benzyl penicillin is extremely soluble in water.

4. False
Penicillin exerts its bactericidal effect by its action on the bacterial cell wall. It prevents the synthesis of the mucopeptide of the cell wall which renders the sensitive organism vulnerable to osmotic pressure.

5. False
Penicillin and the semisynthetic derivatives have no action on the viruses.

5.7   Bacteria resistant to benzyl penicillin include:
1. penicillinase-producing organisms
2. the majority of Gram-negative bacteria
3. Gram-positive anaerobic spore forming organisms
4. the bacteroides
5. *Streptococcus pneumoniae*

1. True
Penicillinase causes a split in the penicillin molecule at the peptide linkage. This destroys the capacity of penicillin to interfere with the synthesis of the bacterial cell wall.

2. True
The majority of Gram-negative bacteria are resistant to the action of

benzyl penicillin because the amount of mucopeptide in their cell walls is considerably less than in the Gram-positive cocci. In addition the greater complexity of the cell wall of Gram-negative organisms hinders penicillin from reaching the site of mucopeptide synthesis. However, some strains of *Escherichia coli, Salmonella typhi* and *Shigella* are sensitive to this drug.

3. False
Both the rod-like spore forming organisms responsible for gas gangrene and tetanus, which are Gram-positive, are sensitive to benzyl penicillin.

4. True
The bacteroides are sensitive only to lincomycin, clindamycin and metranidazole.

5. False
Streptococcus pneumoniae causing lobar pneumonia and the other streptococci responsible for meningitis, otitis media and sinusitis are extremely sensitive to benzyl penicillin.

5.8 Antibiotics which inhibit the synthesis of mucopeptide in the wall of a bacterium include:
1. cycloserine
2. cephalosporins
3. neomycin
4. penicillin and its semisynthetic derivatives
5. erythromycin

1. True
D-cycloserine is a structural analogue of D-alanine and, therefore, effectively inhibits the formation of the dipeptide D-alanyl-D-alanine from D-alanine. This reaction is essential for mucopeptide synthesis and, therefore, the formation of the bacterial cell wall.

2. True
The cephalosporins inhibit the end stages of the synthesis of mucopeptide.

3. False
Neomycin is a bactericidal agent which acts by inhibiting protein synthesis. This antibiotic becomes bound to that part of the ribosomes which absorb transfer-RNA. One theory put forward to explain the action of this and other similar antibiotics such as streptomycin and kanamycin suggests that any messenger RNA molecules which reach ribosomes to which neomycin has become attached are 'misread' in the course of protein synthesis.

4. True
All penicillins act on the end stages of mucopeptide synthesis.

5. False
Erythromycin, a member of the macrolide group of antibiotics which includes sporamycin and oleandomycin, inhibits protein synthesis by mechanisms as yet unknown.

5.9   Ototoxicity is a well recognised complication following the administration of:
1. streptomycin
2. gentamicin
3. neomycin
4. bacitracin
5. erythromycin

1. True
This is the most serious toxic effect of streptomycin. This antibiotic usually causes vestibular disturbance producing vertigo although true deafness occasionally occurs.

2. True
Gentamicin produces labyrinthine damage but this rarely occurs unless renal failure is present. This drug is excreted by the kidney and in the presence of renal failure high serum levels develop even after normal dose schedules, i.e. 80 mg thrice daily. The plasma level of gentamicin should always be monitored especially in patients in whom reduced renal function is known to exist. The dose should be adjusted if the plasma concentration approaches 10–12 ug/ml or if immediately prior to the next injection the level exceeds 2 ug/ml.

3. True
Neomycin can cause irreversible deafness and is the principal reason why this antibiotic is no longer used for systemic treatment.

4. False
This drug is nephrotoxic, not ototoxic. It is not used systemically.

5. False
Erythromycin is exceptionally safe. Erythromycin estolate is hepatotoxic but no other preparations possess this undesirable side effect.

SECTION 6. WOUND HEALING

6.1   Wound healing is enhanced by the administration of:
1. cortisol
2. zinc
3. aldosterone
4. oxygen
5. vitamin C

1. False
Cortisol impairs the synthesis of collagen and enhances its lysis and thus inhibits wound healing.

2. True
Zinc has been shown to accelerate the development of granulation tissue in a wound produced by the excision of a pilonidal sinus. The exact mechanism is unknown but there is evidence that it stabilises macromolecules and stimulates the biosynthesis of collagen.

3. False
Aldosterone has no effect in wound healing.

4. True
The fibroblast requires an ambient pO_2 of around 10 mm Hg in order to synthesize collagen and ground substance.

5. True
Although the administration of vitamin C does not accelerate wound healing a deficiency causes a reduction in the synthesis of collagen and hence a lack of proper healing. If the deficiency of vitamin C is severe and prolonged scurvy develops. In this condition even wounds which have previously healed break down.

6.2   The healing of an incised wound is associated with the following:
1. a lag phase
2. a demolition phase
3. a proliferative phase
4. a contractile phase
5. a maturation phase

1. True
The lag phase in a clean incised wound is a short period during which little cellular activity occurs and the integrity of the wound is maintained by sutures.

2. True
This phase, of minimal duration in a clean incised wound, is associated with the appearance of neutrophils at the margins of the incision which invade the fibrin clot, whilst the cut edges of the epidermis thicken as a result of mitotic activity of the basal cells and, within 48 hours, spurs of epithelial cells from the edges of the wound both migrate and grow along the cut margins of the dermis, fusing to form a continuous but thin layer. By the third day the neutrophils have been largely replaced by macrophages.

3. True
By the fifth day the proliferative phase begins. In this phase great activity of the fibroblast-capillary system occurs which forms a thin layer of granulation tissue between the cut edges of the wound.

4. False
Contraction is an essential feature of an open wound which is healing by secondary union (intention). Precisely how contraction occurs remains unknown although it may be caused by the fibroblasts of the granulation tissue, the myofibroblasts. The magnitude of contraction is greatest in sites where the skin is only loosely attached to the underlying tissues.

5. True
This is the terminal phase of wound healing. During maturation the tensile strength of the wound gradually increases by intermolecular bonding between the collagen fibrils, the wound reaching about 80% of the tensile strength of unwounded skin. In addition the collagen is remodelled in response to mechanical stress placed on the wound.

6.3 The healing of a wound is delayed by:
1. vitamin C deficiency
2. starvation
3. the administration of glucocorticoids
4. lack of blood supply
5. infection

1. True
Wound healing is dependent upon the synthesis of adequate amounts of collagen. This, in turn, is dependent upon the presence of vitamin C. Since man, monkey and the guinea-pig are unable to synthesize this vitamin its absence from the diet disturbs wound healing.

2. True
Starvation will affect wound healing but only when vitamin C deficiency has developed which inhibits collagen synthesis. Otherwise, even in markedly debilitated individuals, normal wound healing takes place.

3. True
The administration of excessive quantities of glucocorticoids causes a defect in collagen synthesis and also diminishes blood vessel formation.

4. True
A deficient blood supply leads to a lack of oxygen in the wound. This in turn diminishes fibroblastic activity because fibroblasts require an ambient O_2 tension of about 10 mm Hg in order to function correctly.

5. True
Infection retards collagen synthesis, enhances the breakdown of pre-existing collagen and hence delays wound healing.

6.4   Collagen, the ultimate source of the strength of a wound:
1. is formed by undifferentiated mesenchymal cells
2. changes with the passage of time
3. undergoes lysis as well as synthesis even when the total collagen content of the wound is remaining constant
4. is broken down by the enzyme collagenase
5. is normally embedded in ground substance

1. False
Collagen is formed in the endoplasmic reticulum of the fibroblasts and excreted into the extracellular space in a monomeric form known as tropocollagen. When its synthesis is disturbed, as for example, in vitamin C deficiency, the precursor material collects and distorts the cell.

2. True
The protocollagen, which is the precursor material excreted into the extracellular space, is hydroxylated under the influence of the enzyme protocollagen hydroxylase. Polymerisation of the tropocollagen also occurs, strong covalent linkages being formed with neighbouring molecules.

3. True
The total amount of collagen in a wound may reach normal levels within 60 to 80 days but qualitative changes occur over a much longer period even though the total amount of collagen in the wound remains practically constant. Lysis is not confined to the wound but extends outwards from it for a variable distance. Should lysis be less intense than synthesis a hypertrophic or keloid scar may develop.

4. True
Collagenase is a naturally produced enzyme which is responsible for the breakdown of collagen. It has been shown in colonic anastomoses that up to 40% of the old collagen is lost in the first 4 to 6 days. This loss of collagen is believed to be responsible for many cases of anastomotic breakdown.

5. True
The collagen fibres are embedded in a ground substance, the chemistry of which is as yet incompletely understood. A major component appears to be large protein-polysaccharide complexes called proteoglycans. Ground substance appears to play a role in the organised precipitation of collagen of which there are 14 different types.

6.5   Post operative infection delays wound healing because:
1. the wound becomes packed with leucocytes
2. many of the organisms involved produce spreading factors which may destroy the intercellular ground substance
3. collagen is destroyed

4. capillary loops fail to develop
5. fibroblasts are diminished in number

1. False
Although the majority of infected wounds become infiltrated with leucocytes these do not delay wound healing. However, if the supply of oxygen is deficient phagocytic function is impaired and their capacity to kill ingested bacteria is diminished.

2. False
Spreading factors do not play a significant role in the delay of wound healing. They are, however, of great importance in the spread of a number of infections particularly gas gangrene.

3. True
Not only does infection lead to the destruction of pre-existing collagen it also retards collagen synthesis. Even in a normal incised wound collagenolysis occurs for a distance of at least 5 mm on either side of the wound and is prominent for about 1 week.

4. False
Capillary loops, essential for the proper function of the fibroblasts, continue to develop in the presence of infection.

5. False
Fibroblasts continue to be produced but the formation of collagen is retarded and collagen which is formed undergoes collagenolysis.

6.6 The following are the features associated with the healing of open wounds:
1. the formation of granulation tissue
2. infection
3. migration of the surrounding epithelium
4. giant cell formation
5. contraction

1. True
Granulation tissue forms during the healing of both clean incised and open wounds, the difference is one of mass, less being formed during the healing of the former than the latter.

2. True
Some degree of infection is nearly always present when an open wound is present. In some circumstances this may be of great significance, e.g. infection of a burn wound by the haemolytic streptococcus may lead to a spreading infection and the destruction of any skin grafts which may be applied.

3. True
Migration of epithelial cells from the surrounding intact epithelium together with their proliferation leads to the formation of a sheet of cells which advances in a series of tongue-like projections beneath any remaining blood clot or exudate on the raw surface of the wound.

4. False
Giant cell formation will not be seen unless foreign material has been buried in the wound. This may then lead to the formation of foreign body giant cells.

5. True
Contraction is an important aspect of the healing of an open wound and it is most conspicuous when the skin is loose. It occurs to a remarkable extent in animals such as the rabbit. The mechanism bringing about contraction is still debatable, but it probably is caused by modified fibroblasts known as myofibroblasts which have an ultrastructure similar to smooth muscle cells. In rabbits, a large wound can be reduced to within 10% of its original size within 6 weeks by contraction.

6.7   Wound healing may be governed by the following:
1. trephones
2. vitamin D
3. chalones
4. mineralocorticoids
5. the availability of sulphur containing aminoacids

1. True
It has been suggested that the stimulus to wound healing is mediated by trephones liberated by damaged cells. Although a working hypothesis based on tissue culture studies, the existence of such substances has yet to be proven in vivo.

2. False
Vitamin D is of little importance in the healing of soft tissue wounds.

3. True
This is a second hypothesis. It has been postulated that normal tissues secrete a substance capable of depressing mitosis, a chalone, and that a wound, by removing some of this depressor substance, permits an increased level of mitotic activity. There is some in vitro experimental work in the rabbit supporting this hypothesis although no chemical substance acting in this manner has yet been identified.

4. False
Mineralocorticoids play no specific part in wound healing but are, of course, of great importance in maintaining the optimal 'milieu interieux' without which normal body functions could not continue.

5. True
The presence of adequate amounts of sulphur containing amino acids such as methionine is essential for collagen synthesis. In well nourished individuals supplementing the diet with extra protein or additional vitamins, especially vitamin C, does not increase the rate of wound healing. The effects of protein and vitamin deficiency only become apparent in the starving animal.

6.8   Woven bone is found:
1. in bone forming in a model of cartilage
2. in fracture haematomas
3. in bones forming in sheets of differentiating mesenchyme
4. replacing lamellar bone in healing fractures
5. surrounding the ends of ununited fractures

1. False
Bone formed in a previous model of cartilage is of a lamellar type. Most of the skeleton is made of lamellar bone which replaces the initial cartilage, hence the term endochondral ossification. Lamellar bone is characterized by the arrangement of the collagen bundles into parallel sheets either forming concentric Haversian systems or flat plates.

2. True
Woven bone with its irregular arrangement of collagen bundles and osteocytes is the first type of bone forming in a fracture haematoma. It is replaced later by mature, lamellar or adult bone which is finally remodelled as the fracture unites.

3. True
Bone formed in differentiating mesenchyme is of the woven variety. This occurs during the embryonic development of the bones of the vault of the skull, the mandible and the clavicle, these bones being referred to as membrane bones.

4. False
The converse is true. Woven bone precedes lamellar bone.

5. False
The ends of ununited fractures are eventually covered by cartilage and if the latter are surrounded by synovial cells a false joint or pseudarthrosis develops. At this stage union becomes impossible regardless of the duration of immobilisation.

6.9   The healing of a closed fracture may be associated with the following pathological consequences:
1. myositis ossificans
2. pseudoarthrosis
3. osteomyelitis
4. osteosarcoma
5. renal calculi

1. True
Immediately following injury a fracture haematoma forms and if the periosteum is torn, blood extends out into the surrounding tissues. Subsequent organisation and ossification leads to the development

of myositis ossificans. This complication is particularly seen following fractures around the elbow joint and the pelvis.

2. True
The mesenchymal cells of the granulation tissue invading the fracture haematoma normally differentiate into bone forming osteoblasts which lay down woven bone. This is later replaced by lamellar bone. If, however, a fracture is imperfectly immobilised these cells may form fibrous tissue, cartilage and finally synovial cells with the result that a false joint develops. This is a well recognised complication of tibial fractures.

3. False
Infection of the fracture site is an extremely rare complication of an uncomplicated closed fracture. It might occasionally occur in patients suffering from multiple injuries in whom a septicaemia develops due to infection elsewhere in the body.

4. False
Although the external callus around the fracture site may lead to a considerable 'tumour' there is no evidence that fractures lead to an increased incidence of osteosarcoma.

5. True
Fractures involving long term immobilisation particularly in the recumbent position may lead to renal calculi. These are often called recumbency calculi and are due to the hypercalciuria which develops in an immobilised patient and the relative stagnation of urine in the lower most calyces of the kidney. In the past, when spinal tuberculosis was relatively common, and prior to the development of antituberculous drugs, such calculi frequently followed the prolonged recumbency necessary to treat the disease.

6.10 Ischaemic necrosis is a recognised complication of fractures of the following bones:
1. talus
2. calcaneum
3. scaphoid
4. pisiform
5. femoral head

The answer is: 1, 3, 5 are **true** and 2 and 4 are **false**.
Ischaemic necrosis following fractures of the talus, scaphoid and femoral head is merely a reflection of the local peculiarities of the blood supply to these bones. Fracture lines running through these bones divorce one fragment from its blood supply with the result that ischaemic necrosis occurs. In fractures of the femoral head the development of ischaemic necrosis leads to pain once weight bearing begins. Radiologically the affected part becomes denser than the surrounding normal bone.

SECTION 7. IMMUNOLOGY

7.1   The following substances normally act as antigens, i.e. stimulate antibody production, when administered to humans:
1. dextrans with a molecular weight below 150 000
2. bovine insulin
3. extracts of Primula
4. human thyroglobulin
5. Rh.D. antigen

1. True
Dextrans are polysaccharides produced by the fermentation of sucrose by certain strains of Leuconostoc mesenteroides. They can be used in the emergency treatment of shock due to a falling blood volume, acting by maintaining the colloid osmotic pressure of plasma. They have no oxygen carrying capacity, contain no plasma proteins or blood clotting factors. Occasionally severe anaphylactic reactions can occur during their administration.

2. True
Insulin antibodies are produced in any diabetic patient treated with non-purified insulin for more than 30 days, in some patients high enough to impair insulin action. Conventional insulins may be separated into: component a, comprising material of high molecular weight, component b comprising pro-insulin, intermediates, a dimer and component c comprising insulin, arginine insulin, the ethyl ester of insulin and desamidoinsulin. It is generally agreed that beef insulin is more antigenic than pork insulin. 'Human' insulin produced by recombinant DNA technology can be produced which is totally non-antigenic.

3. False
Extracts of the Primula have a molecular weight of only 210. They act, however, as haptens binding to the body's own protein through covalent linkages causing them to behave as antigens. This is a common cause of contact sensitivity in gardeners.

4. False
Normally the body does not react against its own thyroglobulin. However, in Hashimoto's thyroiditis autoimmune antibodies make their appearance in the circulation which are directed against thyroglobulin.

5. True
Immunisation with Rhesus antigens occurs in:
(a) Rh negative individuals transfused with Rh +ve blood
(b) In some Rh −ve mothers following a pregnancy in which the fetus is Rh +ve

7.2   The following statements are true or false:
1. IgA is produced at mucous surfaces

2. IgM has a molecular weight of 150 000
3. IgE is the anaphylactic antibody
4. antibody specificity depends on the constant regions of the F(ab) fragment
5. immunoglobulin synthesis is dependent on thymic integrity in neonatal life

1. True

IgA is a very important immunological immunoglobulin frequently secreted as a dimer, Sig A (a compound formed by the combination of two simpler molecules). IgA antibodies are found in secretions covering mucosal surfaces of the stomach and bronchi and in the secretions of the nose, mouth and tears partly bound to high molecular weight mucous.

2. False

IgM has a molecular weight of 970 000. The molecule has a pentameric structure in which each individual heavy chain has a molecular weight of approximately 65 000. The greater part of IgM is within the vascular system and is most frequently seen in the immune response to antigenically complex infectious organisms, e.g. *S. typhi.*

3. True

IgE is the antibody involved in all anaphylactic reactions, binding to the surface of mast cells. An immediate hypersensitivity reaction occurs following the interaction of an antigen (the allergen) with the specific IgE antibody which is predominantly bound to tissue mast cells and circulating basophils. The ensuing reaction results in the mast cells becoming degranulated with the release of mediators producing a variety of effects, e.g. asthma, eczema, hay fever or anaphylaxis, (Type I Hypersensitivity).

4. False

Antibody specificity towards antigen depends on the variable sequence of aminoacids in the adjoining heavy and light chains of the F(ab) fragment of the immunoglobulin molecule.

5. False

Immunoglobulins are secreted by plasma cells of the B-lymphocyte line, cells which are not under thymic control. In birds the site of B-lymphocyte maturation is the Bursa of Fabricus, hence the term B-lymphocyte. This is a lymphoepithelial organ found at the junction of the hind gut and the cloaca. The bursa is colonised by small numbers of stem cells in a few days during early embryonic development and these cells then proliferate and differentiate to form B lymphocytes in the bursal follicles. An equivalent organ has not been identified in mammals, but it has been shown that in neonatal thymectomised mice or children with thymic atresia that although they are unable to produce T lymphocytes, they are still able to produce immunoglobulins.

7.3   Bence–Jones proteins are:
1. the heavy chains of immunoglobulins
2. found in the urine in multiple myeloma
3. associated with a monoclonal gammopathy
4. found in the urine in Waldenström's macroglobulinaemia
5. precipitated by boiling

1. False
Bence–Jones proteins are light chains not associated with the heavy chains which form normal immunoglobulins. They are secreted by the abnormal plasma cells in the condition known as multiple myeloma and pass from the plasma into the urine.

2. True
Bence–Jones proteins are only found in the urine in multiple myeloma. They are a necessary finding for the diagnosis of this disease. Additional diagnostic features of the disease are the presence of osteolytic deposits in the bones and abnormal plasma cells found on sternal marrow biopsy.

3. True
A monoclonal gammopathy together with the presence of an 'M' protein is a necessary feature of multiple myeloma but both are found in other conditions such as old age or following a massive immune response. In the latter conditions they are not associated with Bence–Jones proteins.

4. False
An excess of monoclonal IgM is found in Waldenström's macroglobulinaemia in which, because of the excessive amounts of IgM, the plasma viscosity is increased; a complication which may be reversed by plasmapheresis. Only occasionally does a Bence–Jones proteinuria occur. The clinical features include weakness, fatigue, malaise and anorexia, congestive heart failure, neurological symptoms such as vertigo and nystagmus and occasionally spontaneous haemorrhages from mucosal surfaces. Lymphadenopathy and hepatosplenomegally are common.

5. False
Bence–Jones proteins precipitate at 80°C but return into solution on boiling. Other proteins in the urine are precipitated by boiling.

7.4   T lymphocytes:
1. are immunoglobulin secreting cells
2. are found in the paracortical area of lymph nodes
3. are involved in contact dermatitis
4. are not involved in protection against tuberculosis
5. secrete lymphokines

1. False
T lymphocytes do not produce or secrete immunoglobulins. They carry antibody-like receptor groups on their surface which specifically

react with antigen. These are related to antigen reactive sites on the immunoglobulins as they have the same idiotypes. Anti-idiotypic antibodies produced against immunoglobulin idiotypes react with T lymphocytes responding to the same antigen.

2. True

The paracortical areas of the lymph nodes lie between the true cortex and the corticomedullary junction which is the site of the post-capillary venules with their high walled endothelium. These areas become depleted of lymphocytes in neonatally thymectomised mice and in children born with thymic atresia and because of this the paracortical areas are sometimes known as the thymus dependent areas.

3. True

Contact dermatitis in man is most commonly caused by haptens, molecules too small of themselves to act as antigens, but which conjugated with protein provoke a Type IV hypersensitivity reaction.

Common agents are metals, nickel and dichromate and simple organic compounds such as dinitrochlorobenzene. The process of sensitisation takes between 10–14 days and the reaction once initiated begins to wane after 48–72 hours.

Sensitisation takes place as the hapten-protein conjugate is taken up by the Langerhan cells of the suprabasal epidermis. These cells act as antigen presenting cells and appear in the paracortical areas of the draining lymph nodes in which the T cells are situated. A set of CD4+ lymphocytes are transformed into 'memory' CD4 T cells and then activated CD4 T cells release interferons (INFY) which induce changes in the surface keratinocytes and the endothelial cells of the dermal capillaries, resulting in the liberation of cytokines and the development of an eczematous reaction in the skin.

4. False

Mycobacteria such as *M. tuberculosis* and *M. leprae* are facultative intracellular parasites which tend to reside within macrophages. Host resistance to *M. tuberculosis* is produced by a reaction between specifically sensitised T lymphocytes and mycobacterial antigen. These cells then secrete lymphokines which activate the macrophages causing increased activity of the hexose monophosphate shunt and the intracellular formation of bactericidal superoxides.

5. True

Both T and B lymphocytes will when activated by either specific antigens or mitogenic lectins (carbohydrate binding proteins stimulating cell division) such as phytohaemagglutinin and Concavalin A produce lymphokines; this being the generic term for molecules other than antibodies which are involved in signalling between cells. Such activation can be demonstrated by the development of activation markers which are either an increased expression of existing cell molecules or the de novo appearance of others and by structural changes in the cells which can be seen by both light and electronmicroscopy.

7.5   The major histocompatibility complex (MHC) in man:
1. is situated on chromosome 6
2. has three loci controlling five groups of histocompatibility antigens
3. is involved in the expression of immune response (Ir) genes
4. shows a positive association with Hodgkin's disease, multiple sclerosis and ankylosing spondylitis
5. is tested for by the laboratory on a serum sample

1. True
The major histocompatibility complex consists of four loci situated on chromosome 6 in man. These control four groups of histocompatibility antigens HLA-A, B, C and D. The A and B group of antigens are serologically determined and the D locus antigens are mainly determined by mixed lymphocyte reaction.

2. False
Four loci control four groups of histocompatibility antigens. One antigen in each group is inherited from the father and one from the mother. HLA-D (related) antigens are found mainly on B lymphocytes and these are coded for either by HLA-D or a very closely linked locus. Recently D related antigens have been discovered serologically and are referred to as HLA-DR.

3. True
HLA-D and HLA-DR are considered to be equivalent to the I region of the MHC in the mouse. (Ir) genes coded in this area which are autosomal dominant and inherited in a strictly Mendelian fashion are responsible for the immune response to a number of antigens.

4. True
Hodgkin's disease shows positive association with A1 and B8, multiple sclerosis with A3, B7 and DW2 and ankylosing spondylitis with B8.

5. False
HLA antigens are identified by the use of leucocyte suspensions. The term HLA is an abbreviation of the words human leucocyte antigens. Unclotted blood is needed by the laboratory.

7.6   Macrophages:
1. are not involved in the recognition of antigens
2. do not secrete lysosomal antibodies
3. carry receptors on their surface
4. are involved in the tuberculin reaction
5. play an important role in graft rejection

1. False
Macrophages are important in antigen recognition, immune response genes being expressed by macrophages as well as lymphocytes. The macrophages process antigen which frequently results in the production of a more immunogenic material.

2. False

Following the engulfment of the bacterial cell by the pseudopodia of the macrophage, the bacillus lies in a phagosome. The engulfing macrophage then secretes into the phagosome reactive oxygen intermediates (ROIs), which are toxic to some bacteria and in addition granules and lysosomes fuse with the phagosome pouring into it enzymes which digest the bacterium. Whilst macrophages remain active in the resting state, their function can be enhanced by exposure to lymphokines derived from T cells.

3. True

Macrophages have three distinct forms of receptor:

(1) Fc receptors for IgG with the highest affinity for FcγRL (CD64).

(2) CD14 which is a specific receptor for the lipopolysaccharide capsule of Gram-negative bacteria.

(3) Complement receptors

In addition they have receptors for cytokines which produced by the T cell explains their enhanced activity.

4. True

The tuberculin reaction is an example of type IV hypersensitivity in which following the intradermal injection of tuberculin into an already sensitised individual a skin reaction occurs. In this response, a cellular infiltrate consisting chiefly of CD4+ and CD8+ cells infiltrates the dermis disrupting the collagen bundles. Some 12 hours after the challenge, macrophages begin to accumulate around the dermal vessels, these cells forming the chief antigen-presenting cells stimulating the lymphocytes.

5. False

The important cell in relation to graft rejection is the T lymphocyte. In the absence of these cells, as for example in a mouse in which the thymus has been removed in the neonatal period prior to the release of mature T cells into the periphery, rejection does not occur. Neither B lymphocytes or macrophages play a significant role in primary rejection. Most important in rejection is the action of lymphokines especially IL-2 which is required for the activation of T cytotoxic cells.

7.7 Autoimmunity:

1. occurs because of a breakdown in the ability of the body to distinguish between self and non-self
2. is a rare cause of infertility in the male
3. is not involved in the development of pernicious anaemia
4. is important in the pathogenesis of lupus erythematosus
5. does not result in immune complex disease

1. True

The development of certain human diseases such as Hashimoto's disease of the thyroid is due to a breakdown of the self-recognition mechanisms. The ability to recognise 'self' antigens is determined by the state of maturity of the lymphocyte at the time it encounters the antigen, not as was once thought by the age of the individual. The latter concept arose because it had been shown that if an individual was exposed to a foreign antigen prior to birth, his or her ability to recognise that antigen continued throughout life. However, it is now believed that it is the state of maturity of the lymphocyte and not the individual which is important. When the body is unable to distinguish 'self' and 'non-self', an autoimmune response occurs which results in the development 'autoantibodies'.

Whilst Hashimoto's disease is an organ specific disease, in that only the thyroid gland is affected, there are a range of conditions in which nearly all tissues in the body are affected.

2. True
Rarely infertility in the male is due to the development of antibodies to sperm. As a result the sperms are rendered immobile either by fusing tail to tail or head to head.

3. False
Pernicious anaemia is an autoimmune condition. Normally vitamin B12 is absorbed by the intestine only after it has become associated with the intrinsic factor which is a protein. In P.A. the plasma cells in the gastric mucosa secrete an antibody acting against IF. The resulting lack of vitamin B12 results in the development of pernicious (Addisonian) anaemia which is characterized by the appearance of megaloblastic cells in the peripheral blood. Like many autoimmune conditions, it is commoner in females than in males and frequently runs in families.

4. True
Whereas Hashimoto's disease is an example of an organ specific disease, the autoantibodies being directed solely at the thyroid cells themselves, systemic lupus erythematosus is an example of a non-specific autoimmune disease, in which the autoantibodies are directed against the majority if not all the tissue cells of the body, almost specifically against the cell nucleus.

5. True
Immune complexes are the result of an antigen reacting with antibody. Usually removed by the reticulo endothelial system in some patients in whom the system is defective or overwhelmed, the complexes are deposited in the tissues, e.g. the kidney, joints or skin.

7.8   The germinal centres of lymph nodes:
1. participate in cell-mediated immunity
2. contain macrophages and plasma cells
3. after producing B cells discharge these via the subcapsular (marginal) sinus into the general circulation
4. enlarge in chronic infectious diseases
5. are absent in humans suffering from congenital thymic aplasia

1. False
Cells concerned with cell mediated immunity are not produced in the germinal centres. The germinal centres are concerned with the maturation of B lymphocytes into lymphocyte memory cells and the antibody forming cells. These cells are chiefly concerned with humoral antibody production and develop within the primary nodules in response to antigenic stimulation.

2. True
In addition to proliferating B lymphocytes occasional plasma cells of B lymphocyte origin can be found. In addition macrophages can be seen which contain tangible bodies. These are deeply staining nuclear debris derived from disintegrating cells.

3. False
Lymphocytes enter the lymph node via the afferent lymphatics which give access to the marginal sinus, but cells can only leave the node via the efferent lymphatic at the hilum of the node.

4. True
In chronic infections lymph node enlargement is common because the nodes respond to a number of antigens. In such an enlarged node a characteristic feature is the number of large germinal centres scattered throughout the lymphoid tissue.

5. False
In humans suffering from the rare condition known as the Di George anomaly, organs derived from the third and fourth pharyngeal pouches fail to develop. As a result there is a T-cell deficiency. In addition a variety of facial deformities occur, the eyes are wideset, the ears low and the philtrum of the upper lip is shortened. Because of possible failure of the parathyroid glands to develop, the affected neonate may suffer tetany.

7.9 **Lymphokines, soluble factors released from primed lymphocytes in contact with an antigen are important in:**
1. anaphylaxis
2. immune complex disease
3. macrophage activation
4. graft rejection
5. the involvement of the activation of natural killer cells

1. False
The chief manifestations of anaphylaxis are caused by the degranulation of mast cells with the liberation of a variety of materials such as histamine, platelet activating factors, tryptase and kininogens, together with materials causing smooth muscle spasm such as the leukotrienes and prostaglandins.

2. False
Immune complex disease is also known as Type IV hypersensitivity. Examples include rheumatoid arthritis and glomerulonephritis.

Normally such complexes are removed by the reticuloendothelial system, but if this is ineffective the complexes are deposited in the tissues causing disease.

3. True
Macrophages are activated by a number of lymphokines including interferon-y, granulocyte-macrophage colony stimulating factor (GM-CSF) and tumour necrosis factor (TNFα).

4. True
Lymphokines are an important aspect of cellular rejection. Those particularly involved are IL-2 which activates T cytotoxic cells and IFN4 which induces the MHC antigen expression and also activates macrophages.

5. True
NK cells are activated by lymphokine IL-2. Such cells account for some 15% of the blood lymphocyte population in man and possess many surface markers, a number of which are shared with T cells e.g. CD2 and CD7.

7.10 Antibodies may be detected in vitro by:
1. precipitation
2. complement fixatlon
3. lymphokine production
4. lymphocyte transformation test
5. RIA, ELISA and RAST

1. True
In many cases, if the concentration of antigen and antibody is high enough and at or near equivalence (optimum proportions), the immune complex will precipitate out of solution. This reaction is now performed using agar gel in which cells have been punched and into which the antigen and antibody are separately placed. The solutions diffuse into the gelatin and at the point of meeting, as they bind together, a line of precipitation forms. This can better seen if the gel is washed to remove more soluble proteins and then stained with a protein stain.

2. True
Complement fixation occurs by the classical pathway, i.e. involving C1, C2 and C4 generating C3 convertase, when an immune complex contains IgM and some subclasses of IgG (IgG1 and IgG3), this latter being the major antibody in normal human serum. The fixation of complement can be detected by adding an indicator system such as sheep erythrocytes. If lysis of the RBCs occurs, it indicates that complement is available and has not been used up by the primary system. Conversely if the RBCs remain intact, it indicates that complement has been fixed. Complement fixation is the basis of several diagnostic tests, e.g. the Wassermann reaction and gonococcal complement fixation test and in addition several viral infections.

3. False
Lymphokine is the term used to describe a cytokine produced by a T lymphocyte in cell-mediated immune reactions. Their presence is commonly assayed using their migratory inhibitory properties. In experimental animals peritoneal macrophages and in man, buffy coat leucocytes are used for test purposes.

4. False
The lymphocyte transformation test is based on the proliferative response of specifically sensitised T lymphocytes to an antigen or of T lymphocytes to mitogens such as phytohaemagglutinin or concanavalin-A. It is, therefore, a test of cell-mediated immunity. The proliferative response is assessed by the incorporation of the radioactive nucleoside ^{3}H-thymidine into the cell DNA.

5. True
The technique of RIA, radioimmunoassay and the enzyme linked immunoassay ELISA are all used to defect antigens and antibodies. Using radioallergosorbent test RAST, extremely low concentrations of IgE can be detected. Basically, the technique of RIA requires that the antigen is bound to a plastic plate to which antibody is added, which then binds with antigen. The plate is washed to remove unbound protein, after which the antibody is detected by a radiolabelled binding molecule (the ligand). By using ligands binding only with particular classes of the test antibody, it is possible to distinguish various isotypes. Any unbound ligand is washed away and the radioactivity of the plate is counted on a gamma counter.

7.11 Hypogammaglobulinaemia may occur in the following conditions:
1. prematurity and infancy
2. gluten sensitive enteropathy
3. Di George syndrome
4. autoimmune thyroiditis
5. Hodgkin's lymphomas

1. True
Hypogammaglobulinaemia occurs both in premature and normal infants. Both are protected in neonatal life by maternal IgG, but this is catabolised after birth. Normally, at approximately 3 months of age, normal infants begin to synthesize antibodies, although antibody formation to capsular polysaccharides does not begin until much later. Rarely IgG synthesis is delayed and during this period such infants are susceptible to pyogenic infections.

2. True
Gluten sensitive enteropathy is associated with secondary hypogammaglobulinaemia, due to the disruption of the mucosal lymphoid system (MALT). In this condition the number of plasma cells in the lamina propria decreases with the result that the

concentration of IgA isotype falls, thus reducing the ability of the gut wall to repel bacterial invaders.

3. False
The Di George syndrome is not associated with hypogammaglobulinaemia. This condition is due to a defect in the third and fourth branchial arches during embryonic development. It is not, however, genetically controlled. Thymic dysplasia occurs accompanied by an absence of the parathyroid glands. Humoral antibodies are, therefore, normal in concentration but cell-mediated immunity is defective.

4. False
Autoimmune thyroiditis is associated with an increase in the gammaglobulin levels due to the appearance of a variety of antibodies in the circulation. These react against thyroglobulin, the cytoplasmic components of the thyroid and in approximately 6% of patients, the gastric parietal cells.

5. True
Secondary hypogammaglobulinaemia occurs in Hodgkin's disease, lymphosarcoma, chronic lymphatic leukaemia and tumours of the thymus. Low levels of IgG may also be found in multiple myelomatosis because the neoplastic plasma cells are producing abnormal immunoglobulins.

7.12 Active immunity can be produced by an appropriate vaccine in the following diseases:
1. pneumococcal pneumonia
2. plague
3. chicken pox
4. poliomyelitis
5. typhoid

1. True
Pneumococcal vaccine is a sterile preparation of polysaccharide capsular antigen from 14 serotypes of *Streptococcus pneumoniae*. The commercial vaccine contains 50 μg of polysaccharide from each of the 14 serotypes in 0.5 ml. It should be given to all patients in whom a splenectomy has been performed, since following this operation patients are especially liable to overwhelming pneumococcal septicaemia.

2. True
Plague vaccine is made by producing a sterile suspension of formaldehyde-killed *Yersinia pestis*. One ml of the vaccine contains 3000 million bacteria.

3. False
No suitable vaccine has been prepared which will protect against the pox virus. This is not so for other viral infections, the incidence of

measles; mumps and rubella have all been reduced by using vaccines containing live strains of these viruses. Each vaccine contains a variable number of attenuated organisms which are usually cultured on live chick embryo cells.

4. True
Live attenuated polio virus which can be administered by mouth is now the most commonly used method in the Western World to control this disease. It stimulates the production of antibodies which can be found in the circulation and also produces local resistance in the intestinal tissues by the activation of the MALT system.
In the UK, the trivalent oral vaccine is given; the first dose at three months of age, the second at 6–8 months and a third dose some 4–6 months later.

5. True
The vaccine most commonly used consists of a mixture of cultures of *Salmonella typhi* and *Salmonella paratyphi A, B* and *C* killed by heating at about 60°C and preserved in 0.5% phenol.

7.13 The Arthus reaction:
1. is associated with marked emigration of polymorphonuclear leucocytes into the affected tissues
2. the relative concentration of antigen and antibody is of no importance in this reaction
3. is a delayed hypersensitivity reaction
4. is associated with vascular damage
5. is similar to the Schwartzmann reaction

1. True
One of the major features of the Arthus reaction is the marked polymorphonuclear infiltration which occurs at the height of the reaction. This is in contrast to the infiltration of mononuclear cells accompanying Type IV hypersensitivity reactions such as the tuberculin reaction.
   The PML infiltration is the result of complement activation along either the classical or alternative pathways. In the absence of complement, PML are not attracted to the site. The Arthus reaction reaches a peak in between 4–10 hours following the injection of antigen, after which the PML are replaced by mononuclear cells.

2. False
The relative concentrations of antigen and antibody is of great importance in the Arthus reaction.

3. False
The Arthus reaction is not cell-mediated. It is an example of a Type III hypersensitivity reaction. The reaction reaches a peak between 4–10 hours after the injection of the antigen as compared to the tuberculin reaction, in which the response is maximal between 24–48 hours.

4. True
One of the histological features of the Arthus reaction is the damage to the walls of small blood vessels caused by the liberation of lysosomal enzymes from the polymorphonuclear leucocytes.

5. False
There is no similarity between these two reactions. The Schwartzmann reaction is provoked by the injection of bacterial polysaccharides of the Gram-negative organism, i.e. endotoxin. Schwartzmann himself described how, after the injection of Gram-negative organisms into the skin of a rabbit followed by a second injection given intravenously, haemorrhagic necrosis occurred at the site of the intradermal injection. This is the local reaction. If however the first dose is given intravenously, followed some hours later by a second dose, a systematic reaction occurs in which necrosis of the pancreas, pituitary, adrenals and gut occurs, accompanied by diffuse intravascular coagulation. A sublethal second dose provokes a biphasic fever which after repeated injections is abolished, although the primary pyrogenic effect remains.

7.14 Immune complex disease is associated with:
1. autoimmunity
2. skin graft rejection
3. Pigeon Fancier's lung
4. meningococcal infection
5. talc granuloma

1. True
In both organ specific and non-organ specific autoimmune disease, the clinical presentation is due to failure of the affected individual or animal to deal with the immune complexes formed by the interaction of antigen and antibody. In the human, immune complexes are normally recognised by the mononuclear phagocyte system, particularly in the liver by the Küpffer cells having been transported there bound by CR1 receptors to erythrocytes. If such a process is overwhelmed by the excessive production of complexes, an autoimmune disease follows, e.g. Hashimoto's disease.

2. False
Immune complexes play no part in graft rejection which is a T-cell mediated response, T cells recognising donor-derived peptides in association with the MHC antigens expressed on the graft.

3. True
The basic pathology of Pigeon Fancier's disease is one of an alveolitis in which destruction of the alveoli with associated consolidation occurs due to locally formed immune complexes. The disease follows repeated exposure to pigeon antigens, the antibody induced by such exposure being primarily IgG rather than IgE. When antigen enters the lungs by inhalation, local immune complexes are formed leading to parenchymal destruction.

4. True
Meningococcal infections may be associated with certain stigmata of immune complex disease, such as cutaneous vasculitis, arthritis and episcleritis.

5. False
Talc induces a foreign body granuloma, a non-immunological granuloma, cf. a tuberculous granuloma, distinguished by the absence of lymphocytes. Characteristically the lesion is composed of scattered groups of multi nucleated giant cells, some of which contain the foreign material together with a few macrophages.

7.15 The third component of complement is:
1. a factor in phagocytosis
2. an anaphylatoxin
3. chemotactic
4. a migration inhibition factor
5. an interferon

1. True
Complement C3 gives rise to three products, C3b* (* denotes that this derivation is unstable, interacting chiefly with water and also proteins and sugars), C3c and C3dg which are known as opsonic fragments. The fragments coat the target cells, i.e. bacteria bound by the opsonic receptor sites on the activated phagocytic cells, thus enabling these cells to phagocytose the offending organism.

2. True
An anaphylatoxin is a substance which causes the degranulation of basophils and mast cells with the result that histamine and leukotriene-mediated smooth muscle contraction occurs. Anaphylatoxin activity is present in both the C3a and C5a fractions and an assay of their activity in this regard can be made by observing the contraction of plain muscle in a Schultz–Dale bath. A further effect of anaphylatoxin is to increase vascular permeability accounting for the development of oedema in acute inflammation.

3. True
C3a and C5a are chemotactic to polymorphonucler leucoytes. This explains the Intense polymorphonuclear infiltration which occurs in the Arthus reaction.

4. False
MIF is a group of peptides released by the activation of T lymphocytes which inhibit macrophage migration.

5. False
Interferons are composed of three protein groups IFNα, IFNβ and IFNψ, all of which have an antiviral activity. In addition to this, both IFNα and IFNβ inhibit cell growth and have a possible clinical application in the treatment of some rare malignancies such as renal

cell carcinoma and hairy cell leukaemia. Maximal antiviral activity is shown by IFNα which is produced by leucoytes in response to viruses or nucleic acids.

7.16 Anaphylaxis:
1. develops 24 hours after the initial stimulus
2. causes a weal and flare response
3. is produced by IgA antibody
4. causes eosinophilia
5. causes degranulation of basophilis and mast cells

1. False
Anaphylaxis is an antigen specific immune response classified as a Type I, immediate hypersensitivity reaction. The response is mediated by the specific triggering of IgE sensitised mast cells by an allergen. As a result mast cells become degranulated, leading to either local or generalized effects caused by the liberation of vasoactive amines, of which, in man histamine is the chief effector. Normally exposure to the allergen is followed by a response within minutes.

2. True
If a skin prick test is used to detect Type I hypersensitivity, an immediate weal and flare response follows the injection of the allergen into the skin. The test results in an erythematous and oedematous response vary in severity according to the amount of allergen injected and demonstrates that IgE is bound to the skin mast cells.

3. False
IgA plays no part in anaphylaxis. IgA is present in human serum in which it forms approximately one fifth of the immunoglobulin pool. It is also present in seromucous secretions such as saliva and the secretions of the tracheobronchial mucosa.

4. True
Eosinophils are attracted by products released from T cells, mast cells and basophils known as the eosinophil chemotactic factor of anaphylaxis (ECF-A). These cells release histamine and aryl sulphatase, the latter inactivating the slow reactive substance (SRS-A) of anaphylaxis. However, one of their chief functions is to combat worms and protozoal infections. When a helminth infection of the bowel occurs, T cells recruit eosinophils by means of the Eosinophil Stimulation Promotor (ESP). The eosinophils then adhere to the worm and degranulate, breaking the integument of the worms allowing access to further eosinophils into the body of the worm itself.

5. True
Degranulation of basophil and mast cells follows the interaction between an antigen and IgE. These granules contain heparin and it

is this which stains metachromatically with toluidine blue. The histamine which these cells contain, is formed from histidine by the action of the enzyme histidine decarboxylase; but in addition to histamine, 5-hydroxy tryptamine (serotonin), the slow reacting substance (SRS) of anaphylaxis and basophil derived kallikrein may be released. The latter cleaves the plasma euglobulin kininogen to kinins. The release of these various pharmacologically active agents causes the various local and general manifestations of anaphylaxis.

7.17 Complement activation takes place:
1. in the presence of endotoxin
2. as part of the tuberculin reaction
3. by more than one pathway
4. in anaphylaxis
5. by antigen IgA interaction

1. True
Gram-negative organisms possess an outer coat composed of molecular complexes containing protein, lipid and carbohydrate. Death of the organism, liberates these complexes in the form of endotoxins which are thermolabile at 100°C. When large amounts of endotoxin are liberated by death of the microorganism, endotoxic shock develops which is a response in part mediated by complement. Large quantities of C3a and C5a (anaphylotoxins) are produced, which results in the activation of PML, basophils and mast cells which stimulate intravascular clotting associated with embolisation into the pulmonary microcirculation, producing the clinical syndrome known as 'shock lung'.

2. False
The tuberculin reaction does not involve the complement system. It is a delayed hypersensitivity reaction in which the pharmacological mediators are lymphokines.

3. True
Complement activation resembles the mechanism involved in the clotting of blood, in that it is a cascade reaction which can be activated either by classical or alternative pathways. In all, the complement system consists of some 20 serum proteins, the majority being acute phase proteins, each component reacting with another. In the classical pathway the system is activated by antibodies, IgM, IgG1, IgG2 or IgG3 bound to the surface of a pathogen, whereas in the alternative pathway, the microorganism itself spontaneously activates the complement system by means of its activator surface.

4. False
Anaphylaxis is an antigen-specific immune reaction mediated by mast cells liberating vasoactive materials. This mechanism must not be confused with the action of anaphylotoxins which are complement

peptides C3a and C5a. Anaphylotoxins when injected, cause an anaphylactic reaction by causing mast cell degranulation.

5. False
Although aggregated IgA can activate the alternative pathway under experimental conditions, it is considered that antigen IgA interaction does not normally work through the classical complement cascade.

7.18 The production of antibody is essential to host resistance in the following infections:
1. leprosy
2. *Streptococcus pneumoniae*
3. variola
4. tetanus
5. malaria

1. False
Host resistance to infection with *Mycobacterium leprae* is cell mediated. Three main types of this disease are recognised: tuberculoid, lepromatous and dimorphous or borderline. In tuberculoid leprosy, well defined patches of hypopigmentation of the skin develop, biopsy of which shows an intense lymphocytic and epithelioid infiltration but no microorganisms. In the lepromatous type occurring in patients having a negible resistance to the bacillus, the skin lesions are extremely varied and biopsy shows the presence of numerous bacilli, foamy macrophages and few lymphocytes. Borderline leprosy has the characteristics of both types of lesion. A well known test for leprosy which is of limited value is the lepromin test, in which a cell free filtrate prepared from a ground up excised lepromatous nodule is injected intradermally. The test is of value in following the progress of a patient with borderline disease, because if the initial test is negative and it then becomes positive, it indicates the development of cellular immunity and a swing towards a tuberculoid form of the disease.

2. True
A sterile preparation of polysaccharide capsular antigen from 14 serotypes of *Str. pneumoniae* is now available. These serotypes are considered to be the cause of 80% of all pneumococcal infections. Vaccination by this material is considered mandatory in children in whom a splenectomy has been performed, such children been especially prone to overwhelming infection by this organism.

3. True
Vaccination against variola (small pox) is normally given by applying one dose of a living avirulent vaccine into the skin in the second year of life, complications been least in this age group. The agent used to produce active immunity is a living related virus, known as vaccinia. The vaccine consists of lymph obtained from vesicular lesions produced on the skin of calves or sheep by inoculating the scarified skin with the virus.

4. True

Active immunization against tetanus is achieved by the injection of antigens in the form of tetanus vaccine or the more potent Adsorbed Tetanus Vaccine, this latter consisting of toxoid, a formaldehyde treated product of a growth of *Cl. tetani* which is adsorbed on aluminium hydroxide. A high degree of protection develops of approximately five years duration. Normally three doses are given; 0.5 ml stat, 6–12 weeks later a second dose and a third dose some 6–12 months later still.

5. False

Resistance to malarial infection is dependent of TCD4+ and CD8+ T cells. In malarial infection, an increase in the number of circulating monocytes occurs, together with gross enlargement of the spleen due to an accumulation of macrophages. CD8+ cells destroy infected hepatocytes and also secrete IFNγ which inhibits the multiplication of the *Plasmodium* within these cells. Recently a number of antigens of *Plasmodium falciparum* have been cloned which may in future lead to an effective vaccine.

7.19 Serum sickness:

1. can be caused by an injection of diphtheria antitoxin
2. is common following immunization against tetanus
3. can follow an injection of penicillin
4. is mediated by immune complexes
5. may involve IgE

1. True

Diphtheria antitoxin contains antibodies obtained from the serum or plasma of horses which have been immunized against diphtheria toxin or toxoid. It neutralises circulating toxin but does not affect the pathological changes already induced by the toxin. The cause of the reaction is the formation of antibodies to the horse protein. If the individual has not been previously sensitised, an acute generalized reaction occurs within 7–10 days of the injection, which is clinically characterized by the development of skin rashes, fever, joint pains and frequently swelling of the regional lymph nodes. Both the severity and the duration of the reaction vary greatly. Serum sickness is an example of Type III hypersensitivity.

2. False

Immunization against tetanus is performed by the use of tetanus toxoid. This is a formalised preparation of tetanus toxin which is immunogenic but seldom allergenic, except in persons who are already known to suffer from allergic diseases such as asthma and infantile eczema. If there is such a history, a test dose of 0.2 ml of serum should be injected subcutaneously. If no general reaction occurs over a 30 minute period, the main dose may be given intramuscularly.

3. True
Allergic reactions to penicillin are relatively common. The hypersensitivity is the result of penicilloyl residues from the degradation of penicillin. Prolonged treatment with benzyl penicillin can result in renal failure, biopsy showing tubular damage and an interstitial accumulation of mononuclear cells and eosinophils.

4. True
Serum sickness is an immune complex disease, an example of Type III hypersensitivity which develops in three stages; first the formation of complexes in the circulation, second the deposition of the complexes in various tissues and third an inflammatory reaction provoked by such deposition, due to the activation of complement and the formation of biologically active fragments.

5. True
It is possible that IgE may play a part in Type III hypersensitivity. Induced by the antigen, the IgE antibody may bind to mast cells and platelet activating factors; these mediators then separate the endothelial cells, thus allowing the complexes to enter the vessel wall and then the tissues. Within the tissues, the complexes initiate an acute inflammatory reaction accounting for the joint and renal complications. By immunofluorescent microscopy, the complexes can be seen as granular lumpy deposits of immunoglobulin and complement and, by electron microscopy, as dense deposits along the glomerular basement membrane.

7.20 Anaphylactic reactions commonly follow the administration of the following drugs:
1. penicillin
2. azathioprine
3. procaine
4. α-methyldopa
5. corticosteroids

1. True
Penicillin is an important cause of anaphylactic reactions. The penicilloyl degradation product acts as an hapten binding onto body protein, inducing the formation of IgE antibodies.

2. False
Azathioprine is an immune suppressive and antineoplastic agent with a similar action to 6-mercaptopurine to which it is slowly converted in the body. This agent is an analogue of natural purines. After conversion to active nucleotides including thioinosinic acid, it interferes with nucleic acid synthesis. Azathioprine is chiefly used as an immunosuppressant but it is also used to control certain immune complex diseases, lupus erythematosus, rheumatoid arthritis and chronic active hepatitis. Azathioprine is an antimetabolite which combines with the same enzymes as physiologically occurring cellular metabolites, but prevents the metabolic process.

3. True
Procaine can act as a hapten binding to protein to become an antigen.

4. False
α-methyldopa is an antihypertensive agent classified as an enzyme inhibitor which probably acts centrally. It is now rarely used because of its numerous side effects. In 0.3% of patients to whom methyldopa is administered, an allergic reaction occurs due to the production of autoantibodies similar to warm-reactive antibodies frequently found against Rhesus system antigens. These result in a positive direct Coombs Test.

5. False
The chief side effects of corticosteroids results from disturbances of electrolyte balance, glucogeneogenesis, their adverse action on tissue repair and wound healing and the inhibitory effect on the secretion of corticotrophins by the anterior pituitary resulting in adrenal atrophy. They have no direct immunological effect but, by depressing the activity of PML and reducing the number of circulating lymphocytes, impair the response to acute infections.

7.21 An autoimmune haemolytic anaemia:
1. does not occur in systemic lupus erythematosus
2. does not show Rhesus specificity
3. is associated with a negative Coombs test
4. may be caused by drug therapy
5. is not associated with leucopenia

1. False
Systemic lupus erythematosus is characterized by the development of a large variety of autoantibodies which affect nearly every organ of the body; most are antinuclear. Haematological changes are the commonest clinical manifestation of this condition, of greater frequency than involvement of the joints or skin. Not only are the red cells damaged by autoantibodies, but also by trauma to the red cells in areas of necrotising arteritis and arteriolitis.

2. False
In 30% of patients suffering from a haemolytic anaemia due to 'warm autoantibodies', the specificity of some of these is directed to one or more of the Rhesus antibodies, commonly anti-c or anti-e.

3. False
The major diagnostic criteria of an autoimmune haemolytic anaemia is the positive Coombs test. This test is designed to show the presence of adsorbed antibodies on the surface of red cells. It can be carried out in two ways; either using the patient's own red cells (the direct test) or normal red cells previously mixed with the patient's serum (the indirect test). Anti-human globulin is added to the red cell suspension and causes agglutination when the incomplete antibody is present on the surface.

4. True

Drugs which may be associated with an autoimmune haemolytic anaemia include para-aminosalicylic acid, phenacetin, quinidine, quinine, chlorpromazine, penicillin and α-methyldopa.

5. False

Among the various haematological abnormalities seen in autoimmune haemolytic anaemia, is a leucopenia of less than $4.0 \times 10/L$, a lymphopenia of less than $1.5 \times 10/L$ and a thrombocytopenia of less than $100 \times 10/L$.

7.22 The following are, or contain, autoantibodies:

1. cryoglobulins
2. rheumatoid factor
3. migration inhibitory factor
4. antinuclear factor
5. transfer factor

1. True

Cryoglobulins are immune complexes formed by the reaction between immunoglobulins and anti-immunoglobulin antibodies. Characteristically they precipitate after overnight storage in the refrigerator or when serum is cooled below 37°C. Cryoglobulins are present in the plasma in a wide range of chronic infections and autoimmune diseases, including systemic lupus erythematosus.

2. True

Rheumatoid factor is an IgM anti-immunoglobulin antibody with specificity directed against the Gm groups on the Fc portion of immunoglobulin molecules. It can be detected by the agglutination of latex particles coated with immunoglobulin or by the agglutination of sheep erythrocytes that have reacted with specific rabbit immunoglobulin (Rose–Waaler test). This factor is found in the sera of patients with rheumatoid arthritis and is valuable in distinguishing this disease from the polyarthritis associated with psoriasis. It may also occur, however, in the sera of patients suffering from chronic infections or chronic autoimmune disease.

3. False

The migration inhibitory factor is a lymphokine produced by the action of an antigen or mitogen on T lymphocytes. It inhibits the migration from capillary tubes, in vitro, of macrophages obtained from a peritoneal exudate or leucocytes from the human buffy coat from capillary tubes in vitro.

4. True

The antinuclear factor is an autoantibody directed against DNA and nucleoproteins. It is present in the sera of patients suffering from systemic lupus erythematosus. It may also occur in the sera of patients suffering from chronic infectious diseases such as leprosy and in connective tissue diseases such as Sjögren's syndrome.

5. False
Transfer factor is an extract of human buffy coat leucocytes that can transfer tuberculin sensitivity and other delayed hypersensitivity reactions.

7.23 Antiglobulins may be involved in the:
1. Wassermann reaction
2. Coombs test
3. fluorescent antibody test
4. rheumatoid factor test
5. Casoni test

1. False
The Wassermann reaction is a complement fixation test in which the antigen is cardiolipin derived from ox heart with which the antibody, probably an autoantibody developing in syphilis, reacts. The indicator system used consists of sheep erythrocytes and rabbit (or horse) anti-sheep erythrocyte antibody.

2. True
The direct Coombs test is an agglutination reaction in which erythrocytes coated with antibody are agglutinated by an antiglobulin reagent. The direct Coombs test indicates that sensitised erythrocytes are already present in the circulation as occurs in some haemolytic anaemias. In the indirect test the red cells are sensitised in the laboratory by antibody before exposure to the antiglobulin reagent. This is a very sensitive test for non-agglutinating rhesus antibodies in a patient's serum.

3. True
In the direct fluorescent antibody test fluoroscein may be linked to an antiglobulin through an isothiocyanate linkage. This is then used to detect the presence of bound immunoglobulin fixed in the tissue. Antinuclear factor and other autoantibodies, such as antimitochondrial or antimicrosomal antibodies can be detected by this means.

4. True
Rheumatoid factor is an IgM anti-immunoglobulin molecule that binds to the Gm groups on the Fc portion of the immunoglobulin molecules. It may be detected by the latex agglutination test or Rose–Waaler test. The highest concentrations are found in rheumatoid arthritis.

5. False
The Casoni test is used for the diagnosis of hydatid disease, the causal agent of which is the *Echinococcus granulosus*. In a patient suffering from hydatid disease a local anaphylactic reaction occurs within 15 minutes of the injection of hydatid antigen into the skin with the development of a flare followed by a weal.

7.24 Cell-mediated immunity involves the following mechanisms:
1. IgG
2. T lymphocytes
3. eosinophils
4. complement
5. macrophages

1. False
IgG is an immunoglobulin produced by B lymphocytes. Immunoglobulins are the soluble form of B-cell antigen receptors. IgG plays no part in cell-mediated immunity.

2. True
T lymphocytes are the chief cell concerned in cell-mediated immunity. Lymphocytes developing in the foetal liver and bone marrow develop into T cells in the thymus, due to chemotactic signals emitted from the thymic rudiment. Stem cells reaching the thymus differentiate into thymocytes, which are then able to recognise antigens belonging to the major histocompatibility complex. These antigens are presented to the T cells by a variety of antigen presenting cells.

3. False
Eosinophils are granulocytes in which the bilobed nucleus stains blue with Loishman stain and the cytoplasmic granules red. They comprise between 2–5% of the blood leucocytes in non-allergic individuals. They play no part in cell-mediated immunity, but are especially important in the body's defence against worm infections.

4. False
Complement is an enzymatic system of about 20 serum proteins activated by antigen-antibody reactions; several of the components are acute phase proteins and their chief function is the overall control of inflammation. The system is activated either by the so-called classical pathway or by the alternative pathway.

5. True
Macrophages are concerned with antigen processing and presentation and are the important non-specific effector cell involved in cell-mediated immunity.

7.25 The following tests are based upon a delayed hypersensitivity reaction:
1. Schick test
2. Wassermann reaction
3. Frei test
4. Leishmanin test
5. Prausnitz–Kustner reaction

1. False
The Schick test is used to determine an individual's susceptibility to infection by *Corynebacterium diphtheriae*, the causative organism of

diphtheria which, prior to the Second World War, was the commonest cause of death in children between the ages of 8–10 years in the Western World. To perform the Schick test 0.2 ml of fluid containing a measured dose of diphtheria exotoxin is injected intradermally. A positive red reaction reaching its maximum intensity within 4–7 days signifies a lack of immunity and hence vulnerability to infection. A negative test conversely signifies the presence of antitoxin in the circulation.

2. False

This is a complement fixation reaction used to detect infection with the *Treponema pallidum*, the causative agent of syphilis. In all stages of the disease, immunoglobulins belonging to the IgG and IgM class increase in the serum. To perform the test, antibody i.e. the patient's serum is mixed with complement and antigen and after incubation an indicator system consisting of antibody coated, sheep red cells is added. If complement has been taken up during the incubation stage by the antibody/antigen complex lysis of the added red cells does not occur. Thus a positive CFT is indicated by an absence of lysis. In the Wassermann reaction, the test system consists of the patient's serum in the presence of guinea pig complement.

3. True

The Frei test is a delayed hypersensitivity reaction used in the diagnosis of *L. venereum* which is caused by a specific strain of Chlamydia trachomatis resulting in inflammation of the inguinal and rectal lymph nodes and at the site of the initial infection, a granulomatous ulcer. The causative organism is larger than a virus particle but smaller than a bacterium. The Frei test is performed by the intradermal injection of a heat killed suspension of Chlamydia initially grown on chick yolk sacs. A positive test consists of the development of a swelling at least 7 mm in diameter, reaching a maximum in four days. The test becomes positive 7–40 days after the initial infection.

4. True

The Leishmanin test. Leishmaniasis is an infection of mammals by a protozoa of the genus *Leishmania* with an intracellular stage in the mammalian host and an extracellular flagellate stage in the sand fly. Four species are recognised which cannot be distinguished morphologically. The Leishmanin test indicates the presence of delayed hypersensitivity. A 0.2 ml suspension of promastigotes containing 8×10^6 organisms in 0.5% formal saline is injected intradermally. The reaction is read between 48–72 hours later. When positive, an indurated nodule some 5 mm in diameter develops. If the infection is by *L. donovani*, the Leishmanin test is of no use in diagnosis because the test does not become positive until after recovery from the disease.

5. False

The Prausnitz–Kustner reaction, first described by these two investigators, is an example of Type I hypersensitivity. Kustner was allergic to fish and the injection of his serum into the skin of Prausnitz led to an immediate weal and flare reaction, when fresh antigen was subsequently injected into the skin of the sensitised site. It was later shown that the reaction depended on the formation of IgE immunoglobulin produced by B cells, after an allergen had been presented by antigen presenting cells. It requires cooperation between B cells and T cells and the response is caused by the triggering of IgE sensitised mast cells by the allergen.

7.26 The following are the chief characteristics of delayed hypersensitivity reactions:
1. the development of a polymorphonuclear leucocyte infiltration
2. the reaction has reached its maximum intensity at 4 hours
3. an individual can be passively sensitised with serum
4. it is associated with T-lymphocyte function
5. complement activation is an essential factor

1. False
Polymorphonuclear leucocytes are not involved in any delayed hypersensitivity reactions. The chief cell involved in delayed hypersensitivity is the lymphocyte with the later appearance of the macrophage. In the granulomatous type of delayed hypersensitivity epithelioid cells, possibly derived from activated macrophages and giant cells are found.

2. False
The characteristic feature of all delayed hypersensitivity reactions is that they take more than 12 hours to develop. Even rapidly developing contact dermatitis takes 2–4 days to develop after the application of the offending allergen; this after a period of sensitisation which may require some 14 days.

3. False
Because delayed hypersensitivity reactions are not antibody mediated, passive sensitisation cannot be transferred from one animal to another by serum. In experimental models, however, it can be transferred by sensitised T cells which can be obtained from peripheral blood, lymph nodes or spleen.

4. True
Delayed hypersensitivity follows an interaction between specifically sensitised T lymphocytes and the antigens. In contact hypersensitivity, the hapten forms hapten-carrying complex in the epidermis. Langerhans cells then carry the complex via the lymphatics to the paracortical region of the regional lymph nodes, where interdigitating cells then present the complex to the CD4+ T cells.

5. False
Complement is not involved in the mechanism of delayed hypersensitivity. The equivalent non specific mediators are the

lymphokines. Lymphokine is the generic term for molecules other than antibodies derived from lymphocytes, which are involved in signalling between cells of the immune system.

7.27 Maximum changes occur in the following skin reactions within 24 to 48 hours:
1. Schwartzmann reaction
2. Arthus reaction
3. tuberculin reaction
4. contact patch test
5. skin allograft rejection

1. False
The Schwartzmann reaction is a haemorrhagic reaction in the skin or tissues which reaches its maximum within 4 hours. The local Schwartzmann reaction is elicited in the following manner: an intradermal injection of endotoxin or related polysaccharide is administered followed 24 hours later by an intravenous injection. A generalized reaction involving particularly the lungs and kidneys can be produced if both doses of endotoxin are administered intravenously. It is considered by many investigators that this haemorrhagic reaction underlies similar phenomena observed in bacterial infections such as meningococcal infections in which haemorrhagic destruction of the adrenal glands results in the development of the Waterhouse–Friderickson syndrome.

2. False
The Arthus reaction which is the result of union between antigen and free antibody with the subsequent activation of complement reaches a maximum between 4 and 8 hours. The reaction is chiefly associated with accumulation of polymorphonuclear leucocytes and the aggregation of platelets. Macroscopically the reaction is oedematous and haemorrhagic due to local vasculitis.

3. True
A positive tuberculin reaction occurs following the intradermal injection of tuberculin, a lipo-protein antigen derived from the tubercle bacillus, into a sensitised individual, i.e. an individual already suffering from a tuberculous infection. Following the injection of tuberculin, T cells migrate from the capillaries disrupting the collagen bundles of the epidermis, the reaction reaching a peak after some 48 hours although macrophages, the main antigen presenting cells begin to accumulate around the dermal vessels after approximately 12 hours and increase in density over the ensuing 2–3 days. Unlike contact sensitivity the epidermis does not become oedematous.

4. True
Contact sensitivity was first noticed by Josef Jadassohn in 1886. It is induced by haptens all of which have at least two features in common; a low molecular mass thus allowing the sensitising agent to

diffuse through the skin and an ability to conjugate with the aminoacid side chains of normal body proteins, thus becoming immunogenic and provoking a Type IV hypersensitivity reaction. Common agents are metals, nickel and dichromate and simple organic compounds such as dinitrochlorobenzene. The process of sensitisation takes between 10–14 days and the reaction once initiated begins to wane after 48–72 hours.

Sensitisation takes place as the hapten–protein conjugate is taken up by the Langerhans cells of the suprabasal epidermis. These cells act as antigen presenting cells, and appear in the paracortical areas of the draining lymph nodes in which the T cells are situated. A set of CD4+ lymphocytes are transformed into 'memory' CD4 T cells and then activated CD4 T cells release interferons (INFY) which induce changes in the surface keratinocytes and the endothelial cells of the dermal capillaries resulting in the liberation of cytokines and the development of an eczematous reaction in the skin.

5. False
Although the rejection of a skin graft is also a T-cell mediated immune phenomenon, approximately 10 days are required for rejection in homo sapiens. This is because on primary graft application, it is necessary for the graft to heal and establish a blood supply from the host after which the primary immune response dovolops. This has a latent period of at least 5 days.

7.28 Cell-mediated immune processes are of great importance in the control of the following infections:
1. pneumococcal pneumonia
2. diphtheria
3. tuberculosis
4. candidiasis
5. mumps

1. False
Cell-mediated immunity plays no part in the host's defences against pneumococcal infections. These organisms are opsonised and killed by humoral antibody and complement. The specificity of the antibody is directed against the 'specific soluble substance', the pneumococcal polysaccharide. Antibodies against these soluble antigens were used prior to the introduction of antibiotics for immunotherapeutic purposes with some success.

2. False
Cell-mediated immunity is not involved in diphtheritic infections. *Corynebacterium diphtheriae* is harmful because it produces an exotoxin which particularly damages the myocardium and peripheral nerves. This toxin may be inactivated before it is fixed in the tissues by an antitoxin which can be prepared in the horse. The use of this antitoxin carries the risk of anaphylaxis or serum sickness and, therefore, active immunization with toxoid is preferable.

3. True

Host resistance to mycobacteria is dependent on cell-mediated immune processes. The mycobacteria are facultative intracellular parasites and are found mainly within macrophages. If cell-mediated immunity fails dissemination of the disease occurs and frequently a negative delayed hypersensitivity test is found as in miliary tuberculosis.

4. True

A failure of cell-mediated immunity is frequently associated with mucocutaneous or diffuse candidiasis. Thus diffuse candidiasis may occur in Hodgkin's disease and non-Hodgkin's lymphomas and in the primary T-cell deficiencies of childhood associated with a specific failure of T-cell response to candida antigens. Transfer factor has been successfully used to treat muco-cutaneous candidiasis by specifically increasing the T-cell response to *Candida albicans*.

5. True

Mumps is caused by a paramyxovirus. Previous infection with mumps virus is associated with a positive delayed hypersensitivity skin reaction. Mumps antigen is one of the standard skin test reagents used to diagnose a general non-specific loss of cell-mediated immunity in adults with conditions such as non-Hodgkin's lymphomas, Hodgkin's disease and sarcoidosis.

7.29 The following microorganisms are obligate or falcultative intracellular parasites:

1. *Mycobacterium tuberculosis*
2. *Clostridium welchii*
3. *Corynebacterium diphtheriae*
4. *Leishmania tropica*
5. herpes simplex

1. True

M. tuberculosis may be found within macrophages or other cells of the mononuclear phagocyte series in the centre of a typical epithelioid cell granuloma. *Myco. tuberculosis* requires active cell-mediated immune processes for its elimination.

2. False

Cl. welchii, one of the organisms involved in gas gangrene, is an anaerobic spore bearing organism. The clostridia produce tissue damage by means of exotoxins which are proteolytic and saccharolytic enzymes. In addition the organism produces hyaluronidase which breaks down tissue barriers, thus enabling the organisms to spread through the connective tissue planes. Protection from the clostridial group of organisms may be obtained by the use of an anti gas gangrene serum.

3. False
C. diphtheriae is an aerobic bacillus usually found extracellularly. Its effects are produced by an exotoxin affecting the myocardium and peripheral nerves which can be neutralized by a specific antitoxin.

4. True
The amastigote form of L. tropica, the causative organism of oriental sore, is generally found within macrophages in a granuloma lying within the dermis. In this form the organisms are referred to as 'Leishman-Donovan' bodies.

5. True
Herpes simplex is caused by a virus of the herpes virus group. This group also includes varicella/zoster, the Epstein–Barr virus and cytomegalovirus. Herpes infections are recurrent with long latent periods. Prior to the eruption the virus remains latent in the cells of the posterior root ganglia.

7.30 The following tests may be used to assess host resistance in mycobacterial infections:
1. skin test
2. complement fixation
3. lymphocyte transformation test
4. radioimmunoassay
5. leucocyte migration inhibition test

1. True
The classical way of assessing whether a patient has had previous contact with the Mycobacterium tuberculosis and hence has developed some resistance by means of cell-mediated immunity to the disease is by the tuberculin test. A positive test is indicated by the development over 18 to 48 hours of an inflammatory indurated response in the skin into which tuberculin has been injected. This test is negative during the early stages of infection and in rapidly progressive forms of the disease, e.g. miliary tuberculosis. Similarly the lepromin test conducted with a suspension of Mycobacterium leprae is positive in tuberculoid leprosy but is negative in lepromatous leprosy in which the tissues team with organisms.

2. False
Complement fixation tests are basically used to assess antibody production and since host resistance to mycobacterial infections is cell-mediated these tests play no part in estimating such resistance. Complement fixation tests are used in the diagnosis of viral infections and some bacterial infections such as gonorrhoea and syphilis.

3. True
In this test the patient's lymphocytes are incubated with a mitogen such as phytohaemagglutinin or an antigen to which they have been

primed for some 3 to 5 days. If positive the cells become transformed into large blast cells which readily incorporate ^{3}H-thymidine. This test is used as an in vitro correlate of delayed hypersensitivity and as such frequently correlates well with resistance to infection in conditions in which T cells are important in host protection.

4. False
Radioimmunoassay is used to measure specific IgE antibodies to allergens such as pollens. In the RAST (radioallergosorbent test). It can also be used to measure the concentration of hormones such as insulin in the blood if a specific antiserum is available.

5. True
Buffy coat leucocytes can, under normal circumstances, if cultured overnight, be induced to grow out of the ends of capillary tubes in a fan-like manner. In the presence of antigen and specifically sensitised T lymphocytes, however, migration is inhibited by lymphokine. Such migration inhibition correlates with delayed hypersensitivity and host resistance in mycobacterial infections.

7.31 The following cells play an important role in skin allograft rejection:
1. polymorphonuclear leucocytes
2. macrophages
3. mast cells
4. B lymphocytes
5. T lymphocytes

1. False
Polymorphonuclear leucocytes play no part in skin allograft rejection. These cells play their major role in acute inflammatory reactions and immunological reactions mediated by immune complex deposition, such as the Arthus reaction.

2. True
Skin allograft rejection is a T-cell mediated event in which lymphokine is released. The latter is the generic name given to soluble factors released by primed lymphocytes after contact with a specific antigen. These substances are chemotactic for macrophages and cause the activation of macrophage enzymes. Macrophages form the major cellular component of the mononuclear infiltrate which develops around a skin allograft prior to rejection.

3. False
These cells play no part in skin allograft rejection. They are of particular importance, however, in anaphylactic reactions when degranulation results in the liberation of the vasoactive amines, histamine, serotonin, SRS-A and kallikrien. Degranulation is initiated by the interaction between antigen and IgE antibody on the cell membrane.

4. False
The B lymphocytes are the precursors of plasma cells which produce immunoglobulins. The latter are not considered to play a major role in skin graft rejection. B lymphocytes, which are not so mobile as T lymphocytes, are found chiefly in collections in central lymphoid tissues, i.e. the spleen and lymph nodes, particularly in the lymph follicles, germinal centres and at the cortico-medullary junction.

5. True
Skin allograft rejection is a cell-mediated event caused by the reaction of specifically sensitised T lymphocytes with antigen. The T lymphocytes are part of the mobile pool of long-lived lymphocytes which may be found circulating through the tissues and in the lymph. They migrate into the tissues particularly through post-capillary venules. The production of lymphokine by reaction with antigen brings the next most important cell, the macrophage into the area of activity.

7.32 The following substances are lymphokines:
1. properdin
2. migration inhibitory factor
3. macrophage chemotactic factor
4. Factor B
5. interferon

1. False
Properdin is a β globulin found in normal serum. It is part of the complement alternative pathway to C3 conversion by-passing C1, C4 and C2. It is activated by bacterial endotoxins and polysaccharides such as zymosan which is obtained from yeast and insulin. Mg^{++} but not Ca^{++} ions are necessary for the activation of the alternative pathway.

2. True
The migration inhibitory factor (MIF), a glycoprotein with a molecular weight of approximately 40 000, was the first of the various substances now known under the generic title of lymphokines to be discovered. It is assayed by its ability to inhibit the migration of macrophages obtained from the peritoneal exudate of the guinea-pig from capillary tubes in vitro.

3. True
Macrophage chemotactic factor is another lymphokine. It is distinguished from the polymorph chemotactic factor by its molecular weight. It is assayed by its ability to attract macrophages onto a millipore membrane in a closed Boyden chamber.

4. False
Factor B is an important component in the alternative pathway of complement activation. It is also referred to as C3 proactivator.

5. True
Interferons are a family of substances, molecular weight approximately 30 000, produced by cells infected with a virus or by synthetic inducers such as polyinosinic and polycytidylic acid (poly I:C). They can also be produced by T lymphocytes activated by antigen or mitogen and as such are included in lists of lymphokines. When taken up by other cells interferon inhibits the replication of virus within them.

7.33   Graft versus host disease:
1. may follow bone marrow transplants
2. may follow blood transfusion
3. occurs in Hodgkin's disease
4. can be suppressed by tetracyclines
5. can be suppressed by cyclophosphamide

1. True
Bone marrow transplants are used as a therapeutic measure in patients suffering from the combined immunodeficiency syndrome or whose immune response has been destroyed by irradiation or cytotoxic drugs. If the marrow transplant is not HLA matched the donor T lymphocytes will react against host tissues. Signs that this is occurring include the development of erythroderma, exfoliative dermatitis, splenomegaly and wasting. Death ultimately occurs if the reaction cannot be controlled by immunosuppressive agents such as cyclosporin A.

2. True
In patients suffering from a severe depression of their immunological systems a blood transfusion may provoke a graft versus host reaction due to the T cells which are contained in the donor blood. This can be avoided by irradiating the blood prior to transfusion in order to destroy T-cell function.

3. False
Graft versus host disease could only occur in a patient with Hodgkin's disease if that patient was rendered completely immunodeficient by irradiation or cytotoxic therapy and then received a transfusion of unirradiated blood.

4. False
Tetracyclines will only suppress the intercurrent infection that occurs as the graft versus host reaction becomes severe and then only if the bacteria causing the infection are sensitive to this antibiotic. This is not usually the case since the common agents of infections in this disease are fungi and viruses, all of which are insensitive to the tetracyclines.

5. True
Temporary suppression of the graft versus host reaction can be achieved by the use of cyclophosphamide because this drug is a nitrogen mustard derivative cytotoxic to dividing lymphocytes. It is,

however, an extremely toxic compound which may cause hair loss resulting in alopecia, destruction of the bladder mucosa causing haematuria and increasing susceptibility to fungal infection.

7.34 The following can cause immunological unresponsiveness:
1. immunological tolerance
2. immunological enhancement
3. Freund's adjuvant
4. T lymphocytes
5. antigen-antibody complexes

1. True
Immunological tolerance is the term given to the specific immunological unresponsiveness caused by the elimination or depletion of a specific clone of immunologically competent cells. This may be the result of exposure to high concentrations of antigen, particularly in late fetal or early neonatal life which is the period of immunological immaturity. This phenomenon is mainly applicable to allograft rejection.

2. True
Immunological enhancement paradoxically does not refer to the enhancement of the immune response but to enhancement of tumour growth. This is caused by the stimulation by the tumour of a blocking antibody which combines with the antigenic sites on the surface of the tumour cells. This results in a markedly decreased stimulation of cell-mediated immunity against the tumour and also prevents the sensitised T cells reacting with tumour antigens to kill the tumour cells.

3. False
Freund's adjuvant is a water in oil emulsion with or without added mycobacteria. The addition of antigen to this mixture promotes both increased antibody formation and delayed hypersensitivity.

4. True
A special subpopulation of T lymphocytes may act as suppressor cells diminishing the immune response. In mice these cells can be distinguished by the presence of surface antigens (Ly antigens) from the effector cells of delayed hypersensitivity and helper cells required both in vitro and in vivo for antibody formation.

5. True
The presence of soluble antigen-antibody complexes formed between soluble tumour antigens and antibody in the circulation can suppress the cell-mediated immune response against tumours and lead to enhanced tumour growth.

7.35 The following infections are common in immunodeficient patients:
1. *Pneumocystis carinii*

2. diphtheria
3. poliomyelitis
4. cytomegalovirus
5. *Candida albicans*

1. True
Pneumocystis carinii is a protozoan related to the plasmodia and toxoplasma. It is ubiquitous in the upper respiratory tract but causes chronic pneumonia in patients who have become immunodeficient whether due to malnutrition, the administration of cytotoxic drugs in the treatment of Hodgkin's disease or primary T-lymphocyte deficiency.

2. False
There is no evidence that an increase in infection by *Corynebacterium diphtheriae* occurs in immunodeficient subjects.

3. False
There is no evidence of an increase in infection with poliovirus occurring in immunodeficient subjects.

4. True
Cytomegalovirus is a herpes virus causing cytomegalic inclusion disease. Although infection with this virus is commonly associated with the newborn it is also an important opportunistic infection occurring in immunodeficient patients. The virus affects many tissues and intracellular inclusion bodies are found particularly in the bronchial epithelium.

5. True
Mucocutaneous candidiasis is a particular complication of immunodeficiency regardless of the cause. It is generally associated with other evidence of depressed T-lymphocyte function, negative candidin skin test, depressed lymphocyte transformation test and absent leucocyte migration inhibition test with candida antigens. Other non-specific tests of T-lymphocyte function may also be depressed.

7.36 The following conditions are associated with T-cell immunodeficiency:
1. Hodgkin's disease
2. Tay–Sachs disease
3. Wiskott–Aldrich syndrome
4. Down's syndrome
5. Di George syndrome

1. True
The pathological tissue in Hodgkin's disease permeates the T-lymphocyte areas of lymphoid tissue, the B lymphocytes and plasma cells remaining unaffected. Many of the tests of T-lymphocyte function (skin tests, mitogen induced lymphocyte

transformation) become depressed as the disease progresses. Patients become susceptible to opportunistic infections with organisms normally controlled by T-lymphocyte function, including *Pneumocystis carinii*, cytomegalovirus, *Candida albicans* and other fungal agents.

2. False
Tay–Sachs disease is a lipid storage disease affecting the nervous system only. The ganglion cells are ballooned with ganglioside giving rise to amaurotic familial idiocy. These children typically have a cherry red spot in the macula.

3. True
This is a sex linked recessive disease manifested in childhood in which there is delayed growth and thrombocytopenia, the platelets being both small in number and abnormal in structure. Such children develop severe eczema and pyogenic infections. The serum contains increased amounts of IgA and IgE, normal levels of IgG but T-cell function is defective and cell-mediated immunity becomes progressively worse so that affected children become susceptible to viral, fungal and bacterial infections.

4. False
Down's syndrome, once known as mongolism, is associated with trisomy of chromosome 21. This chromosomal abnormality gives rise to mental retardation as well as the characteristic physical features. Although there may be an increased incidence of leukaemias it is not associated with immunodeficiency.

5. True
The Di George syndrome is due to a defect in development of the third and fourth branchial arches resulting in thymic aplasia and T-cell immunodeficiency, together with an absence of the parathyroid glands which causes hypocalcaemic tetany.

7.37   A non-specific depression of the tuberculin reaction occurs in:
1. influenza
2. measles
3. sarcoidosis
4. leprosy
5. ulcerative colitis

1. False
Infection with the influenza virus does not lead to non-specific depression of cell-mediated immunity.

2. True
The depression of tuberculin reactivity in measles was first described by Von Pirquet in 1908 and it was eventually established that this was the result of infection of the T-lymphocytes with the virus. The disease is frequently accompanied by a lymphopenia. The

lymphocyte transformation and leucocyte migration inhibition responses to tuberculin and candida antigens are lost.

3. True
Certain parameters of T-lymphocyte function are depressed in sarcoidosis including the tuberculin reaction and ability to cause sensitisation with 2.4 dinitrochlorobenzene (DNCB). In addition, the lymphocyte transformation response in the presence of phytohaemagglutinin (PHA) may be depressed.

4. True
A non-specific depression of tuberculin reactivity and the ability to be sensitised with DNCB occurs in over 50% patients with lepromatous leprosy but only occasionally in tuberculoid leprosy. However, there is no generalized decline in T-lymphocyte function which apart from the specific loss of cell-mediated immunity against *Mycobacterium leprae* is otherwise normal.

5. False
There is no evidence of even a partial loss of T-lymphocyte function in ulcerative colitis and tuberculin reactivity remains therefore within normal limits.

7.38 Haptoglobins
1. bind to the body's own proteins to make them immunogenic
2. are immunoglobulins
3. bind to free haemoglobin
4. are controlled by genetic factors
5. can bind rheumatoid factor

1. True
Haptens are simple chemical groupings that are too small to be immunogenic, but can interact with antibody. They can bind to proteins generally by covalent linkages to become immunogenic.

2. False
Haptoglobins are α_2 globulin glycoproteins with a molecular weight not exceeding 1000. They carry only one or two antigenic determinants.

3. True
Haptoglobins bind to free haemoglobin.

4. True
Three types of haptoglobin can be distinguished by the use of electrophoresis. Each type is determined by the interaction of two co-dominant somatic genes Hp^1 and Hp^2.

5. False
Haptoglobins play no part in the rheumatoid factor. The latter is an autoantibody directed against the Gm antigens on the heavy chain of IgG molecules. Gm antigens form allotypes of immunoglobulin

molecules. This characteristic of IgG molecules is determined by a dominant autosomal gene.

SECTION 8. DISORDERS OF THE PLASMA PROTEINS

8.1   The total plasma protein level is low in:
1. patients suffering from protein-losing enteropathy
2. patients suffering from cardiac failure associated with oedema
3. oedema due to the nephrotic syndrome
4. nutritional oedema
5. patients suffering from chronic liver disease

1. True
Normally the gut accounts for less than 10% of the total protein degradation. However an increased output of protein may occur in a variety of conditions:
  (a) From disorders of the intestinal lymphatics leading to loss of lymph into the gut
  (b) Inflammatory or ulcerative conditions of the intestines such as Crohn's disease and ulcerative colitis
  (c) specific conditions affecting the stomach:
     (1) Mènétrier's disease in which there is a profound hyperplasia of the surface mucous cells with accompanying glandular hypertrophy
     (2) Gastric gland hyperplasia secondary to excessive gastrin secretion as in the Zollinger–Ellison syndrome, caused by gastrinoma.

2. False
Hypoproteinaemia does not occur or play any part in the oedema associated with cardiac failure. The protein content of oedema associated with congestive heart failure is that of a typical transudate. The specific gravity is low, the protein content is less than 10 g/L and no fibrinogen is present. The oedema of cardiac failure is partially due to the rise in venous pressure and partially to an increased vascular permeability caused by the poor blood flow.

3. True
The nephrotic syndrome is associated with a massive proteinuria. In adults a daily loss in excess of 3.5 g of protein may occur leading to plasma levels of less than 3g/dl with the result that generalized oedema follows due to the fall in colloid osmotic pressure. In addition an associated sodium and water retention due to a compensating secretion of aldosterone occurs. Basically the proteinuria is caused by a derangement of the glomerular capillary walls resulting in an increased permeability to plasma protein.

4. True
Chronic severe lack of protein may lead to nutritional oedema, the deficient uptake of aminoacids impeding the formation of albumin by

the cells of the liver. The consequent fall in the colloid osmotic pressure is the chief contributory cause of oedema developing, but in addition as, in the nephrotic syndrome, sodium and water retention plays its part. Clinically the oedema is unrecognisable until the interstitial fluid volume has increased by some 10% above the normal level. In such circumstances pitting is observed.

5. True
In severe cirrhosis the number of hepatocytes is decreased and those remaining may have a reduced functional capacity. All albumin in the body is synthesized by the liver cells in zones which electronmicroscopy shows contain rough surfaced endoplasmic reticulum rich in ribosomes. In addition to failure to produce albumin, the movement of protein from the hepatocytes into the circulation may be impaired by collagenisation of the Space of Disse into which, under normal circumstances, the abundant microvilli of the hepatocytes protrude.

8.2   The nephrotic syndrome is associated with:
1. no evidence of sodium retention
2. high levels of aldosterone in the urine
3. high levels of antidiuretic hormone in the urine
4. an increased blood volume
5. hypolipidaemia

1. False
Both sodium and water retention are associated with the nephrotic syndrome due to a biochemical chain reaction which includes a compensatory increase in the secretion of aldosterone mediated by the hypovolaemic enhanced antidiuretic hormone secretion, stimulation of the sympathetic system and a reduction in the secretion of natriuretic factor such as atrial peptides.

2. True
As a result of increased secretion of aldosterone, abnormally high levels of this hormone are found in the urine.

3. True
The secretion of the antidiuretic hormone which in mammals is a nonapeptide, arginine vasopressin, is increased due to the reduction of the total or effective blood volume.

4. False
The blood volume is diminished in the nephrotic syndrome due to the low plasma protein level which reduces the colloid osmotic pressure.

5. False
The majority of patients suffering from the nephrotic syndrome have a hyperlipidaemia due to an increase in circulating cholesterol, trigylcerides, very low density lipoproteins (VLDL), low density lipoproteins (LDL) and lipoprotein (a). The precise cause remains to be established but may be due to an increased synthesis of

lipoproteins by the liver cells, abnormal transport of circulating lipid particles and decrease catabolism. Lipuria follows the hyperlipidaemia because lipoproteins leak across the glomerular capillary wall. The lipid appears in the urine as free fat or 'oval fat bodies' which represent lipoprotein reabsorbed by tubular epithelial cells and then shed.

8.3   Secondary hypogammaglobulinaemia occurs in:
1. sarcoidosis
2. congestive heart failure
3. malnutrition
4. chronic lymphatic leukaemia
5. nephrotic syndrome

1. False
Sarcoidosis is normally associated with an increase in IgG particularly in cases with active extensive disease. It is accompanied by a depression of cutaneous delayed hypersensitivity. Patients exhibit a negative tuberculin test, but if cortisone is injected with tuberculin antigen the skin test becomes positive, the converse of what would normally be expected.

2. False
Hypogammaglobulinaemia does not occur in association with the oedema of congestive heart failure.

3. True
Protein-calorie malnutrition also called protein energy malnutrition or PEM, is associated with a functional defect in both the B and T lymphocytes leading to secondary hypogammaglobulinaemia and decreased immunoglobulin synthesis.

4. True
In at least half the cases of chronic lymphatic leukaemia there is a reduction in all classes of immunoglobulin. In early cases only IgM may be reduced.

5. True
Protein loss due to failure of reabsorption from the renal tubules can cause a depression of the serum immunoglobulins as well as albumin.

8.4   A monoclonal gammopathy occurs in the following diseases:
1. lepromatous leprosy
2. kala-azar
3. multiple myeloma
4. lymphatic leukaemia
5. active chronic hepatitis

1. and 2. False
In both leprosy and kala-azar a specific defect in T-lymphocyte

immunity to the infecting organism is present. The result is a widespread dissemination of the organism throughout the skin, as in lepromatous leprosy, or organs as in systemic leishmaniasis. These forms of disease are associated with negative delayed hypersensitivity tests to antigens from the infecting organisms but B-lymphocyte function is not affected and consequently high levels of antibody to the infecting organism are present. An associated generalized polyclonal increase in immunoglobulin synthesis also occurs.

3. True
Multiple myeloma is a plasma cell malignancy originating in the bone marrow involving both the skeleton and extraosseous sites. The disease is caused by the expression of a single clone of immunoglobulin secreting cells, the plasma cells, and as a result a single homogeneous immunoglobulin is produced. The monoclonal immunoglobulin identified in the blood is referred to as an M compound in reference to myeloma. It has a molecular weight of 160 000.

4. True
Chronic lymphatic leukaemia accounts for some 25% of all cases of leukaemia, occurring usually over the age of 50, affecting males twice as commonly as females. It is a neoplastic disorder of B lymphocytes which express Ig (IgM and IgD) but the number of immunoglobulin molecules is so low they may appear to be sIg negative by immunofluorescence. They express λ or κ light chains indicating monoclonality.

5. False
Active chronic hepatitis is associated with a polyclonal increase in immunoglobulins, anti-nuclear factor, rheumatoid factor and anti-mitochondrial and antismooth muscle autoantibodies. As well as liver involvement there may be other evidence of immunological disease such as arthritis.

8.5 The following conditions are associated with a polyclonal gammopathy:
1. Waldenström's macroglobulaemia
2. rheumatoid arthritis
3. Down's syndrome
4. Wiskott–Aldrich syndrome
5. post-streptococcal glomerulonephritis

1. False
Waldenström's macroglobulinaemia usually presents between the sixth and seventh decade with a group of non-specific symptoms such as fatigue, weakness and weight loss, although in 50% of patients a lymphadenopathy, hepatomegaly and splenomegaly are present. Pathologically the bone marrow is diffusely infiltrated with

lymphocytes and plasma cells which synthesize a monoclonal IgM immunoglobulin leading to a macroglobulinaemia which causes a greatly increased viscosity of the blood.

2. True
Rheumatoid arthritis is a chronic inflammatory disorder which may affect many tissues. Its most obvious and usual presentation is the occurrence of joint disease in which a proliferative synovitis results in destruction of the articular cartilage and ultimately in severe cases ankylosis of the affected joints. Approximately 80% of patients suffering from the disease develop autoantibodies to the Fc portion of the autologous IgG and IgM.

3. False
There is no evidence of increased immunoglobulin synthesis in Down's syndrome which is a genetic defect associated with three instead of the normal pair of number 21 chromosomes.

4. False
The Wiskott–Aldrich syndrome is a condition in which atopic eczema, thrombocytopenia and an increased susceptibility to infection in infants occurs. It is a sex linked recessive condition accompanied by a defect in antibody production, low levels of IgM and defective T-cell function.

5. True
Acute post-streptococcal glomerulonephritis occurs most frequently in children between 6 and 10 years of age. It is caused by certain strains of Group A beta-haemolytic streptococci, chiefly types 12, 4 and 1. A latent period of some four weeks occurs after the streptococcal infection, usually of the throat or skin during which antibodies and immune complexes are formed, the latter being deposited in the mesangium and the basement membrane of the glomeruli at which points immunofluorescent microscopy shows granular deposits of IgG, IgM and C3.

SECTION 9. DISORDERS OF CALCIUM METABOLISM

9.1   The normal level of ionised calcium in the plasma is maintained by the following mechanisms:
1. the secretion of calcitonin
2. the presence of 1,25 $(OH)_2 D_3$
3. parathyroid hormone secretion
4. renal tubular conservation
5. the circulating level of magnesium

1. True
Calcitonin is a small polypeptide hormone secreted by specialized 'C' cells which in the mammalian thyroid are derived embryologically

from the ultimobranchial organs. The only known physiological regulator of the rate of calcitonin secretion is the concentration of Ca ion in the plasma and extracellular fluid. The chief functions of calcitonin are to regulate calcium homeostasis and bone remodelling. The sensitivity of the human to changing calcium levels is related to age; CT is a much more effective hypocalcaemic agent in the young than the old.

2. True
$1,25 (OH)_2 D_3$ is the active metabolite of vitamin D3. Vitamin D3 is the natural form of vitamin D in man and is synthesized in the skin from 7-dehydro-cholecalciferol by a photochemical reaction. If because of social factors this process is blocked, the deficiency must be made good by dietary intake. The rate of conversion is determined by the plasma calcium level which exerts its effect indirectly by altering the ratio of secretion of PTH and CT. The major functions of vitamin D are to increase the retention of calcium and PO4 and secondly to control the mineralisation of bone.

3. True
The two chief target organs of PTH are the kidney and bone. An increase in PTH secretion by the parathyroids increases the plasma Ca concentration and decreases the PO4 concentration and in addition it increases the urinary excretion of phosphate and hydroxyproline-containing peptides.

4. True
An increase in the level of circulating PTH decreases the urinary secretion of calcium. Approximately 247 000 mmol of calcium are filtered through the glomeruli in a day, but renal conservation is so complete that only 1% is daily excreted in the urine. This is due to the action of PTH on the distal nephron.

5. False
Changes in the level of circulating magnesium can occur without the serum calcium level altering. However, hypomagnesaemia may occur in hyperparathyroidism and PTH increases the renal tubular reabsorption of magnesium.

9.2 Hypercalcaemia is associated with:
1. increased excitability of the neuromuscular apparatus
2. band keratitis
3. metastatic calcification
4. a prolonged Q–T interval
5. renal stones

1. False
Hypocalcaemia causes increased excitability of the neuromuscular junctions, thus giving rise to the two classical signs known as Trousseau's sign, induced carpopedal spasm on reducing the circulation to the arm by means of a blood pressure cuff and

Chvostek's sign, a twitch of the facial muscles following a sharp tap over the facial nerve. Hypercalcaemia is associated with decreased excitability, about twice as much galvanic current being required to excite a peripheral nerve as in the normal state. This probably accounts for the generalized muscle weakness which can occur in primary hyperparathyroidism.

2. True
A form of keratitis known as band keratitis occurs in hypercalcaemia from any cause.

3. True
Metastatic calcification is the deposition of calcium in normal tissues (cf. dystrophic calcification in which calcification takes place in abnormal tissues). Metastatic calcification takes place in any condition in which hypercalcaemia occurs, hyperparathyroidism, vitamin D intoxication and the milk-alkali syndrome. The most common sites are the interstitial tissues of blood vessels, kidneys and lungs. The deposits may be amorphous or as hydroxyappatite crystals.

4. False
The Q–T interval is shortened in any condition in which hypercalcaemia develops; a prolonged Q–T interval is a significant finding in hypocalcaemia.

5. True
Renal stones either composed of calcium oxalate or calcium oxalate/phosphate occur in hypercalcaemia. Calcium oxalate stones occur in 5% of patients suffering from hypercalcaemia, although in about half the patients suffering from this type of calculus hypercalciuria will be present in the absence of hypercalcaemia.

9.3 The destruction of bone is associated with the following biochemical changes:
1. an increased secretion of hydroxyproline in the urine
2. an elevated alkaline phosphatase
3. an elevated acid phosphatase
4. an elevated serum calcium
5. depression of the serum phosphate

1. True
When bone collagen is destroyed most of it is hydrolysed to its constituent amino acids which are then re-used or degraded further to carbon dioxide and urea. However, 5-8% of collagen is only partially degraded into soluble hydroxyproline-containing peptides which circulate in the blood stream and are excreted in the urine.

2. True
Serum alkaline phosphatase comes from three sites: liver, bone and intestine. In normal subjects liver and bone contribute almost equal

amounts and the contribution by the intestinal mucosa is small. In conditions causing bone destruction the alkaline phosphatase rises. However, a similar rise also occurs in liver diseases, particularly in biliary cirrhosis. A distinction between liver and bone disease is possible if the concentration of enzymes such as leucine aminopeptidase which is only produced by the cholangioles is determined.

3. False
This enzyme is synthesized in the prostate and its level is usually elevated in the presence of a malignant prostate particularly if skeletal secondaries are present. Both the alkaline and acid phosphatases may be raised in this situation because typical prostatic secondary deposits are associated not only with destruction but also the laying down of new bone, producing osteoplastic or sclerotic metastases.

4. True
The level of the serum calcium rises in the presence of severe bone destruction, e.g. when generalized osteolytic bone deposits are present leading to hypercalcaemia and metastatic calcification particularly in the kidney.

5. True
The relationship between calcium and phosphate is reciprocal. Any condition, such as bone destruction, which raises the circulating level of calcium is normally associated with a depression of the phosphate concentration.

9.4 Hypercalcaemia and hypercalciuria is caused by:
1. osteolytic secondary deposits in bone
2. hypervitaminosis D, often referred to as vitamin D intoxication
3. parathyroid adenomata or carcinomata
4. tumours of adrenal medulla
5. primary carcinoma of the kidney

1. True
All osteolytic secondary deposits cause hypercalcaemia and hypercalciuria because of the breakdown of bone and the liberation of calcium.

2. True
The administration of excessive quantities of vitamin D leads to an increase in calcium absorption from the gut and hence an increase in the blood calcium followed by hypercalciuria. Given in excessive amounts over a prolonged period, irreversible renal damage may occur due to the development of nephrocalcinosis.

3. True
Benign or malignant tumours of the parathyroids or simple hyperplasia results in an increase in the concentration of circulating

parathyroid hormone. This causes a variety of effects on the cells found in bone including:

(a) The activation of adenylcyclase in the osteoblasts
(b) Stimulation of osteoclast division

The net result is increased bone resorption associated with hypercalcaemia and hypercalciuria.

4. False
Tumours of the adrenal medulla secrete noradrenaline and adrenaline which have no effect on the skeleton or the serum calcium.

5. False
The only hormone secreted by the kidney is erythropoietin which is one of the many factors controlling the production of red cells. This hormone is produced by the action of an enzyme-like factor on a plasma substrate. The regulation of the rate at which erythropoietin is produced is determined by the relationship between the oxygen supply to the kidney and the metabolic needs of that organ.

9.5   Excessive osteoid tissue is found in:
1. vitamin D deficiency
2. Muslim women
3. patients on anticonvulsant drugs
4. patients on long-term anticoagulant therapy
5. long-standing obstructive jaundice

1. True
A deficiency of vitamin D in adults impairs or blocks the normal mineralisation of osteoid laid down in the remodelling of bone, producing osteomalacia. In growing children, there is also inadequate provisional mineralisation of epiphyseal cartilage leading to rickets. This effect is mediated by the defective absorption of calcium from the gut leading to hypocalcaemia.

2. True
Muslim women may have a relatively high incidence of osteomalacia in which excessive osteoid occurs in the skeleton because their extensive clothing prevents vitamin D_3 synthesis from 7-dihydrocholesterol by ultra violet light.

3. True
Several anticonvulsant drugs, of which phenytoin is an example, if given for prolonged periods may lead to the excessive formation of osteoid. This is probably due to the stimulus these drugs give to the production in the liver of isoenzymes which convert vitamin D to inactive metabolites.

4. False
Long term anticoagulant therapy has no effect on vitamin D synthesis or bone development.

5. True

The absorption of vitamin D requires the presence of bile salts, absorption normally occurring in the lower part of the small intestine. The vitamin is then hydroxylated in the liver and altered in the kidney to its biologically most active form. A vitamin D deficiency is, therefore, theoretically possible in long standing obstructive jaundice.

9.6   The sites in which metastatic calcification occurs are:
1. the kidney
2. the wall of the inferior vena cava
3. old tuberculous lesions
4. atheroma
5. the cornea

1. True

In pathological conditions associated with hypercalcaemia and hypercalciuria, calcium is deposited in the tubular epithelial cells causing cellular damage. Calcified cellular debris then blocks the tubular lumen causing an obstructive atrophy of the nephrons with interstitial fibrosis. Atrophy of the entire cortical areas drained by the damaged tubules may occur leading to cortical scarring. The earliest functional defect is an inability to elaborate a concentrated urine.

2. False

Calcification is rare in the walls of veins, possibly because of the high CO_2 content of venous blood and the low pH.

3. False

The calcification which occurs in old tuberculous lesions is dystrophic calcification. It occurs in tuberculous lesions because of the high fat content of caseous pus. This is due to the high lipid content of the *M. tuberculosis* which is liberated from the bacillus when it dies.

4. False

Calcification certainly occurs in atheromatous plaques but this is also dystrophic in nature. Calcium is deposited because of the high concentration of lipid in atheroma.

5. True

The cornea is frequently affected and the condition can be discovered during life by slit lamp examination.

9.7   Osteoporosis differs from osteomalacia in that:
1. the radiographic density of the skeleton is reduced in the former and not the latter
2. the remaining bone in the former presents a normal histological appearance
3. major changes occur in the epiphyses in the former
4. pseudofractures are commoner in the former than the latter
5. excess osteoid tissue is present in the former

1. False

This is one of the cardinal changes in both conditions. It is a reflection of the decrease in the mass of calcified bone. In osteomalacia usually due to vitamin D deficiency, there is a derangement of the mineralisation of bone, osteoid is laid down but is not calcified. In osteoporosis the bone mass is reduced. This is a normal age related phenomenon approximately 0.7% of bone being lost per year after the attainment of the peak bone mass in young adult life.

2. True

Osteoporosis, commonly observed following the menopause, is associated with a decrease in the total amount of bone, although the cellular composition of the remaining bone is normal as is the degree of mineralisation. Two general theories have been advanced to account for the development of osteoporosis, a decreased rate of new bone formation or enhanced bone resorption. Additional factors are the diminishing function of the osteoblasts with increasing age and in postmenopausal women oestrogen deficiency.

3. False

Changes in the epiphyses are characteristic of osteomalacia if its onset occurs before the epiphyses fuse as in rickets. Osteomalacia is caused by vitamin D deficiency and is associated with a failure of mineralisation of the osteoid and the cartilage of the epiphyseal growth plate in childhood. Radiological examination of affected long bones shows wide, irregular fuzzy, cupped metaphyses, thin bony cortices and the late appearance of epiphyseal centres.

4. False

Whilst fractures are common in established osteoporosis, pseudofractures, otherwise known as Looser's zones are characteristic of osteomalacia. Radiologically they are radiotranslucent lines which lie either at right angles or obliquely to the cortical outlines of the bones and often traverse them. They are commonly bilateral and symetrical and are most frequently found in the axillary margins of the scapula and the neck of the femora.

5. False

Excess osteoid is the characteristic feature of osteomalacia. Calcification, however, fails to occur in the absence of vitamin D.

9.8   Urinary hydroxyproline excretion may be increased in:

1. Paget's disease of bone
2. Cushing's syndrome
3. hypopituitarism in children
4. hyperthyroidism
5. extensive fractures

The answers are:

1. True

2. False
3. False
4. True
5. True

When collagen is destroyed it is first degraded into soluble peptides containing the amino acid hydroxyproline. Most of the hydroxyproline is then degraded into carbon dioxide and urea but a small percentage circulates in the plasma to be excreted in the urine. Although the relationship between hydroxyproline excretion and bone resorption is not as simple as first appeared elevated values are normally taken as evidence that such a change is taking place.

In normal circumstances 8 to 10% of the hydroxyproline in the dietary gelatin and collagen appears in the urine and in addition recently synthesized collagen also contributes to the total urinary hydroxyproline.

In Paget's disease, which is a primary disorder of skeletal remodelling, the rapid turnover of bone leads to high urinary levels of hydroxyproline whereas in Cushing's disease attrition of the bone matrix leads to generalized osteoporosis. Weakening of the vertebral bodies produces bulging of the intervertebral discs giving rise to the classical radiological appearance of 'codfish' vertebrae but no rise in the urinary hydroxyproline value occurs because the bone matrix remains normal.

9.9   The following conditions may be described as metabolic bone disease:
1. osteoporosis
2. Paget's disease
3. osteomalacia
4. osteopetrosis
5. osteitis fibrosa cystica

1. True
Albright defined metabolic bone disease as one in which a generalized disorder of bone arises as a consequence of a disturbance in general body metabolism. All bones are therefore involved although some may exhibit more pronounced changes than others. Osteoporosis fits into Albright's definition since there is an overall loss of bone mass even though that remaining retains its normal cellular appearance and degree of mineralisation.

2. False
Paget's disease is not a metabolic bone disease. It is a condition of unknown aetiology, although possibly due to a slow virus infection caused by a paramyxovirus in which periods of osteoclastic activity are followed by bone formation. In about 15% of patients only a single bone is involved. In the remainder the condition is polyostotic chiefly involving the pelvis, spine and skull. The affected bone is typically enlarged with thick coarsened corticoid and cancellous bone.

3. True
This change is accompanied histologically by decreased mineralisation and the presence of excess osteoid. Radiologically typical changes occur in the epiphyses as in rickets and in many patients pseudofractures known as Looser's zones occur. These are linear zones of translucency, cutting across at right angles to and usually affecting only one cortex.

4. True
This is a hereditary disorder characterized by osteoclast dysfunction resulting in diffuse symetrical skeletal sclerosis. The bones become grossly thickened and lack a medullary canal. The bone which is formed is not remodelled and tends to be woven so that the bone becomes brittle. Owing to the absence of the medullary cavity, extramedullary haemopoiesis causes hepatosplenomegaly.

5. True
Radiological examination of the bone in this condition shows cyst formation and areas of bone erosion. Histologically the affected bone shows marked osteoclastic activity and secondary fibrosis. Microfractures followed by haemorrhages occur, producing the so-called 'red bone tumours' due to the fibrous tissue and the deposition of haemosiderin.

SECTION 10. OEDEMA AND AMYLOID

10.1 Oedema occurs in:
1. Cushing's syndrome
2. Conn's syndrome
3. Zollinger–Ellison syndrome
4. Klinefelter's syndrome
5. pregnancy

1. True
Cushing's syndrome is caused by the excessive secretion of both mineralo- and gluco-corticoids by the adrenal cortex, due to hyperplasia, an adenoma or a malignant tumour. Sodium retention follows, with the result that oedema develops. Additional factors are the associated hypertension and a chemical change of the interstitial tissues allowing more fluid retention.

2. False
Conn's syndrome or primary hyperaldosteronism is associated with a cortical adenoma or bilateral zona glomerulosa hyperplasia. It normally presents with either hypertension or the symptoms of hypokalaemia (muscle weakness or paralysis). Sodium and water retention occurs which causes the hypertension, but oedema does not develop because of increasing sodium excretion by the kidneys.

3. False
The Zollinger–Ellison syndrome is caused by hyperplasia, benign adenoma or a malignant tumour of the D cells of the pancreas. This results in the secretion of large amounts of gastrin which in turn stimulates the parietal cells causing them to secrete acid at their maximal capacity. So great is the output, that the pH of the upper jejunum may be less than 2 at which point pancreatic lipase is inactivated and bile salts may be precipitated causing steatorrhoea. The pathological result of the excessive acid secretion is usually multiple ulceration which may develop in abnormal situations.

4. False
This syndrome is not associated with oedema. It is one of the commonest chromosomal disorders resulting from the presence of a Y chromosome together with a second X, the Y chromosome ensuring the formation of the testes and masculine development but the second X preventing the development of the testes.

5. True
Pregnancy is associated with fluid retention which thus gives rise to oedema particularly in the dependent parts. In late pregnancy hypertension and pre-eclampsia may lead to worsening of the condition.

10.2 Angioneurotic oedema is associated with:
1. depression
2. complement deficiency
3. immunoglobulin E
4. menstruation
5. NSAID poisoning

1. False
Although the term 'angioneurotic' may suggest an underlying psychiatric disorder, this is not so. The term is used to describe an oedema, mainly of an urticarial type which is frequently seen on the face and neck. The more recent term to describe the condition is angio-oedema.

2. False
Complement is normal in angio-oedema but in the hereditary form which is an autosomal dominant condition there is a deficiency of Cl inhibitor. This permits complement activation to go unchecked and the mast cells to degranulate, liberating vasoactive peptides. In this condition sporadic attacks particularly affecting the face and gut occur.

3. True
Urticarial angio-oedema is relatively common in atopic children, the term used to describe 10–15% of the population who suffer from allergic disorders including angio-oedema, asthma, eczema and food allergies. The development of the angio-oedema follows the

ingestion of food allergens and is mediated by IgE. The IgE causes the degradation of mast cells with the release of vasoactive amines.

4. False
The salt and water retention associated with the premenstrual period are normally not associated with increased capillary permeability and oedema.

5. False
The common clinical features of poisoning with non-steroidal anti-inflammatory agents are nausea and vomiting, gastrointestinal haemorrhage, headache, tinnitus, disorientation, confusion and haematuria associated with renal failure. Hepatic dysfunction can also be caused together with a metabolic acidosis.

10.3 Pulmonary oedema may occur in patients suffering from:
1. major trauma
2. plague
3. right-sided heart failure
4. hypoproteinaemia
5. nematode infections

1. True
Patients suffering from multiple injuries may develop the condition of 'shock lung', now more commonly known as ARDS, Adult Respiratory Distress Syndrome. Initially there are few if any pulmonary symptoms but these usually develop within 48 hours. Even when the patient is complaining of dyspnoea and tachycardia, the appearance of the chest x-ray may be normal. Later as pulmonary oedema develops, patchy infiltrates appear. These develop due to an increase in capillary permeability due to a variety of factors including cytokines, oxygen radicals, complement and arachidonate metabolites.

2. True
Pulmonary oedema is a pathological facet of pneumonic plague caused by *Yersinia pestis*, a Gram-negative falcultative intracellular bacterium transmitted by flea bites. The major pulmonary pathology is the development of a severe confluent haemorrhagic and necrotising bronchopneumonia.

3. False
Pulmonary oedema occurs in left-sided heart failure and is most commonly seen in patients suffering from a failing heart due to hypertension, aortic valvular disease or following a myocardial infarct. The clinical manifestations in the early stages occur at night, causing attacks of nocturnal dyspnoea (cardiac asthma).
Pathologically fluid initially accumulates in the basal regions of the lower lobes because hydrostatic pressure is greatest in these areas. Histologically the alveolar capillaries are engorged and haemosiderin-laden macrophages (heart failure cells) may be seen.

4. False

Hypoproteinaemia does not specifically cause pulmonary oedema except as a terminal event when cardiac failure occurs. However, hypoproteinaemia is associated with peripheral dependent oedema.

5. False

Nematode larvae of ankylostomes and ascaris may migrate through the lungs and cause pulmonary eosinophilia. This may be associated with pneumonic consolidation but there is no evidence that they cause pulmonary oedema.

10.4 Amyloid is deposited most frequently in:
   1. liver
   2. brain
   3. spleen
   4. lungs
   5. kidneys

1. True

Amyloidosis of the liver is not necessarily associated with hepatomegaly. The material is first seen in the Space of Disse and then progressively encroaches into the adjacent hepatic parenchymal cells and sinusoids causing progressive deformity and pressure atrophy. The cut surface of the liver has a waxy refractile appearance. Despite advanced disease, liver function is not usually severely impaired.

2. True

Although the CNS is not usually affected by amyloidosis, a condition known as amyloid angiopathy is almost invariably found in Alzheimer's disease, immunohistological staining for amyloid beta-peptide showing the deposition of amyloid in the walls of the smaller cortical vessels.

3. True

Amyloid deposits in the spleen take two forms. In one the Malpighian bodies are changed into translucent globules by amyloid deposition in their reticulum, hence the term sago spleen, in which splenomegaly is not marked. In the other form the change affects the reticulum of the red pulp, the walls of the venous sinuses and many of the small arteries. In this latter type the spleen may be palpable and weigh up to 1 kg; this is a rarer condition than the sago spleen and is only common in tertiary syphilis.

4. False

The lungs are an infrequent site of amyloid deposition although deposits may occur in primary amyloidosis, i.e. amyloidosis occurring in the absence of any predisposing cause.

5. True

Renal amyloidosis is particularly important because once established, renal failure is almost inevitable and indeed renal amyloidosis is the most frequently recorded cause of death. The kidneys may be of normal size, enlarged or lastly shrunken owing to the deposition of amyloid within the arterial and arteriolar walls. The initial deposits of amyloid appear in the glomeruli causing distortion but the interstitial peritubular tissue, arteries and arterioles are also affected. Involvement of the capillaries makes them more permeable to albumin, causing a heavy proteinuria leading to the nephrotic syndrome.

10.5 The following conditions are particularly associated with the deposition of amyloid:
1. gas gangrene
2. leprosy
3. chronic osteomyelitis
4. Type II diabetes
5. pneumococcal pneumonia

1. False
Secondary amyloidosis is a feature of chronic rather than acute infections.

2. True
Secondary amyloidosis is a frequent cause of death in lepromatous leprosy, resulting from the renal failure caused by the renal deposition of amyloid. In contrast amyloidosis is not a particular feature of tuberculoid leprosy.

3. True
Secondary amyloidosis occurs in chronic pyogenic osteomyelitis when the fibril is amyloid A (AA) and the related serum protein is serum amyloid A (SAA). AA amyloid is identical in all patients and is derived from the aminoterminal two thirds of an acute phase protein (SAA) which is synthesized in the liver as an apoprotein. SAA levels may increase a 1000 fold during an inflammatory response.

4. True
In Type II or non-insulin dependent diabetes amyloid consisting of a 37-aminoacid peptide known as amylin is found in the islets. It has been suggested that the amyloid in this situation is secreted by the hyperfunctioning B cells in parallel with insulin. This type of diabetes is not the result of failure to secrete insulin but resistance on the part of the individual to the action of insulin, this resulting in constant hyperfunction of the B cells.

5. False
Acute pneumococcal pulmonary infections as with all acute infections do not lead to amyloidosis.

10.6 Secondary amyloidosis occurs in the following conditions:
1. familial Mediterranean fever
2. thalassaemia

3. sickle-cell disease
4. multiple myeloma
5. rheumatoid arthritis

1. True
This is a rare genetic disorder largely restricted to Armenians,
Sephardic Jews and other ethnic groups in the Middle East.
Inheritance is normally autosomal recessive. Clinically the disease is
characterized by recurring joint and abdominal pain and fever. It
frequently presents in childhood and each attack may last 12–72
hours, but the attacks may be very intermittent. Amyloid fibrils
biochemically resembling AA are deposited in the kidneys leading to
proteinuria and finally renal failure.

2. False
This is a haemoglobinopathy occurring in the Mediterranean region.
Amyloid does not develop but the condition is complicated by
haemosiderosis and cirrhosis of the liver.

3. False
Sickle-cell disease is another haemoglobinopathy causing chronic
anaemia. Attacks of 'sickling' may be precipitated by dehydration,
chilling and infection. An attack is normally associated with severe
pain. The complications include ulceration of the legs, respiratory
infection, cardiomyopathy and thrombotic crises.

4. True
In multiple myeloma, renal involvement may be the result of the light
chains (Bence–Jones) proteins, the light chains being toxic to the
tubular epithelial cells or by the deposition of paraprotein either in the
form of alpha or kappa light chain fragments in the blood vessels of
the glomeruli and tubules resulting in renal failure. The most frequent
paraprotein in multiple myeloma is a monoclonal IgG.

5. True
Rheumatoid arthritis has now replaced chronic pyogenic infection as
the commonest cause of secondary amyloidosis. Postmortem
examination reveals amyloid deposits in 20% of all cases. This
disease is of unknown aetiology but with many immunological
features including circulating IgM anti-immunoglobulin antibodies
(the rheumatoid factor).

10.7 The essential constituents of primary amyloid include:
1. immunoglobulin
2. complement
3. albumin
4. starch
5. fibrils

1. True
Two distinct types of amyloid are recognised, primary and
secondary. In primary amyloidosis, the amyloid is derived from

plasma cells and consists of AL protein made up of complete immunoglobulin light chains, the NH2-terminal fragments of light chains or both. In secondary amyloidosis, the amyloid protein (AA) does not have the structural homology to immunoglobulin, the AA fibrils are derived from a larger protein precursor in the serum called SAA (serum amyloid-associated protein) which is synthesized in the liver and circulates in association with a sub-group of lipoprotein. In both types, the major component of the fibrils (95%) is amyloid material and the remaining 5% is known as P component, which is a glycoprotein very similar in composition to a C-reactive protein (an acute phase reactant).

2. False
The complement proteins are not components of amyloid.

3. False
Albumin is not a component of amyloid.

4. False
The term amyloid was first used by Virchow in 1842 because it stained violet with iodine after treatment with sulphuric acid, in the same way as starch. The most widely used stain for amyloid is Congo red which under ordinary light microscopy imparts a pinkish/red colour to the deposit. When observed by polarising microscopy, the deposits appear green.

5. True
In all forms of amyloid, whether primary or secondary, the basic structure is that of non-branching fibrils of indefinite length and with a diameter of approximately 10 nm. X-ray crystallography demonstrates a characteristic cross pleated configuration regardless of the clinical condition or its chemical composition.

10.8 Amyloidosis may be associated with elevated levels of the following serum proteins:
1. β-lipoprotein
2. SAA
3. IgD
4. M-protein
5. β-microglobulin

1. False
Amyloidosis is not associated with elevated serum levels of β-lipoprotein. An elevation of these components occurs in a number of familial conditions and may lead to atherosclerosis with its attendant complications.

2. True
SAA (serum amyloid-associated protein) circulates in association with HDL 3 subclass of lipoprotein. It is from SAA that AA amyloid associated protein is derived, AA being a nonimmunoglobulin protein

synthesized in the liver under the influence of cytokines. It is raised in all cases of secondary amyloidosis.

3. False
IgD is present in low concentration in the serum. Increased levels of IgD may occur in chronic infections or in IgD myelomas.

4. True
M protein is found in increased amounts in the serum of patients suffering from plasma cell neoplasms. The malignant B cells synthesize abnormal amounts of a single specific immunoglobulin (monoclonal gammopathy) producing an M (myeloma) protein spike on electrophoresis.

5. False
$\beta 2$ microglobulin is a peptide which is a non-polymorphic protein in man which is a part of the HLC antigen.

10.9 Amyloid reacts with the following stains:
1. thioflavine-T
2. fluoroscein isothiocyanate
3. methyl violet
4. methyl green
5. Congo red

1. True
Thioflavine–T is a fluorochrome which reacts with amyloid. It is particularly useful for demonstrating small glomerular deposits.

2. False
Fluoroscein isothiocyanate does not stain amyloid deposits. It is used to conjugate with antibody in the fluorescent antibody technique.

3. True
Methyl violet is a metachromatic stain, staining normal tissue violet and amyloid pink.

4. False
Methyl green does not stain amyloid deposits. It reacts specifically with DNA and is used as part of the methyl green-pyronin stain (Unna–Pappenheim) which is specific for DNA and RNA.

5. True
The Congo red test for amyloid depends on the specificity of this dye for amyloid. Intravenously administered Congo red disappears rapidly from the circulation in amyloid disease due to its rapid conjugation with this material. Amyloid material stained with Congo red can be seen to best advantage when the tissue is examined in polarised light when a green birefringence can be seen. Biopsy material to establish the presence of amyloid is usually taken from the rectum, gums or kidney.

SECTION 11. PIGMENTATION

11.1 Generalized pigmentation of the skin occurs in:
1. carcinoma of the head of the pancreas
2. idiopathic hereditary haemochromatosis
3. argyria
4. arsenic poisoning
5. black liver disease

1. True
One of the first clinical manifestations of carcinoma of the head of the pancreas may be the onset of jaundice due to increasing compression of the common bile duct. The colour of the skin tends to be olive green due to the retention of biliverdin. Removal of the obstruction does not result in an abrupt return to normal due to the strong affinity of elastic tissue for bile pigments.

2. True
Idiopathic hereditary haemochromatosis is one of the commonest inborn errors of metabolism, transmitted as an autosomal recessive, the gene being located in the short arm of Chromosome 6. Excessive dietary iron absorption takes place and is stored as haemosiderin or ferritin. Symptoms develop when about 20 g of stored iron has occurred. The metal is stored in the liver eventually causing micronodular cirrhosis, in the interstitial tissues of the heart causing heart failure and in the pancreas both in the exocrine and islets leading to diabetes, and in the joints. Disruption of the islets results in diabetes hence the alternative name for the condition of 'bronzed diabetes', from the slate grey pigmentation caused by the accumulation of haemosiderin in the dermal macrophages and fibroblasts.

3. True
The prolonged administration of remedies containing silver preparations is followed by the deposition of brownish granules of silver compounds in the skin, gut wall and basement membrane of the glomeruli and renal collecting tubules.

4. False
Chronic exposure to arsenic leads to gastrointestinal upset, weakness, weight loss and muscle pains. Individuals who recover from arsenical poisoning commonly develop peripheral neuropathy, desquamation of the skin and hyperpigmentation and hyperkeratosis of the palms and soles of the feet.

5. False
This is a synergistic infection found in sheep in which *Cl. oedematiens* is frequently harboured in the liver in the absence of disease. Should the animal become infected with the liver fluke, *Fasciola hepatica,* the local conditions created favour the growth of

the clostridia and the animal develops a condition known as black liver disease.

11.2 Patchy skin pigmentation occurs in the following conditions:
1. Peutz–Jeghers syndrome
2. familial polyposis
3. Addison's disease
4. purpura
5. vitiligo

1. True

The Peutz–Jeghers syndrome is an autosomal dominant disease. The external marker of the condition is patchy circumscribed circumoral and intraoral melanotic pigmentation. The chief importance of the condition, however, is the development of harmatomatous polyps which are chiefly situated in the small bowel causing intermittent attacks of small bowel colic due to the intussusceptions which they provoke. However, in about one third of all patients similar polyps are found in the stomach and large bowel. This type of polyp has no malignant potential but there is an overall increased frequency of carcinoma of the pancreas, breast, ovary and uterus in sufferers of this condition.

2. False

Pigmentation does not occur in familial polyposis or the related condition known as Gardner's syndrome, in which latter the large bowel polyps are associated with sebaceous cysts, osteomata of the face and skull and desmoid tumours.

3. False

Addison's disease, due either to a chronic destructive disease of the adrenal by tuberculosis or to an autoimmune phenomenon, is typically associated with a generalized pigmentation of the skin due to the excessive release of melanocyte stimulating hormone by the anterior pituitary due to the decline in adrenal inhibition. The hyperpigmentation particularly affects areas of the skin exposed to the sun, pressure points such as the elbows and knees and the knuckles.

4. True

Any cause of purpura or bruising leads to temporary localized staining of the skin. This is due to the dermal macrophages retaining some of the iron released from the red cells and incrustation of the collagen molecules with iron.

5. False

Vitiligo is a patchy macular form of depigmentation caused by loss of melanocytes; compare this to albinism in which melanocytes are present but melanin is not produced because of a defect in tyrosinase. Vitiligo may be an autoimmune condition, a view supported by the presence of circulating antibodies to melanocytes.

11.3   The following endocrine abnormalities lead to generalized pigmentation:
1. Cushing's disease
2. Carcinoid tumours
3. Zollinger–Ellison syndrome
4. Addison's disease
5. Sheehan's syndrome

1. True
Cushing's disease is associated with high plasma ACTH levels. This hormone possesses melanocyte stimulating properties although it is not as potent as MSH.

2. False
Although the face and upper chest may be cyanotic in colour and bright red flushes occur in this syndrome there is no true pigmentation. The flushes are provoked by alcohol and may be inhibited by α-adrenergic blocking agents.

3. False
This syndrome in which a gastrin secreting tumour of the pancreatic islet cells occurs is not associated with pigmentation. A common presenting syndrome is intractable duodenal ulceration.

4. True
Addison's disease follows destruction of the adrenal glands. This leads to very high outputs of ACTH and MSH leading to melanin deposition and striking hyperpigmentation. The agent responsible is believed to be beta-MSH which is an extremely potent pigmentary hormone. The plasma concentration of this hormone is roughly parallel to the degree of hyperpigmentation.

5. False
Sheehan's syndrome is the commonest cause of non-neoplastic spontaneous hypopituitarism in the adult female. It arises from destruction of the anterior pituitary in females who suffer from a postpartum haemorrhage associated with shock. The exact mechanism by which the gland is destroyed is unknown, but during pregnancy the pituitary enlarges to almost twice its normal size compressing the blood supply. Sudden hypotension is thought to precipitate spasm of the vessels causing ischaemic necrosis of most, if not all of the anterior lobe. Contributory factors may be the development of disseminated intravascular coagulation or the presence of concommitant disease such as sickle cell anaemia. If the patient recovers, rapid mammary involution and failure of lactation occurs which are the earliest recognisable signs. This is followed by chronic debility and eventually hypothyroidism. The skin becomes pale due to loss of melanin and dry. A loss of axillary and pubic hair also occurs.

11.4   Hereditary or idiopathic haemochromatosis is:
1. more common in the female than the male

2. an autosomal recessive disorder
3. associated with a material staining with Congo red
4. complicated by malignancy
5. associated with arthritis

1. False
Males predominate in a proportion of 5:1 because the physiological loss of iron by menstruation delays the accumulation of iron.

2. True
HHC is a homozygous recessive hereditary disorder leading to the continuous accumulation of iron throughout life, usually between 0.5–1 g/ annually.

3. False
The classic stain used to detect iron in the tissues is potassium ferrocyanide and hydrochloric acid, the Prussian blue reaction.

4. True
Iron accumulates in the liver, not only in the heptocytes but also in due course in the bile duct epithelium and Küpffer cells. In due course, micronodular cirrhosis develops and later still hepatocellular carcinoma which is one of the commonest causes of death in this condition.

5. True
The deposition of haemosiderin in the synovium may cause an acute synovitis.

11.5 Haemosiderosis differs from haemochromatosis in that:
1. the former is more common in the Bantu
2. the latter is due to the excessive absorption of iron and the former to excessive intake
3. in the former the excessive iron is chiefly deposited in the parenchymal cells, whereas in the latter the excess iron is deposited chiefly in the macrophages of the liver, spleen and bone marrow
4. in the former cirrhosis does not develop
5. in the latter the level of plasma transferrin is abnormally high

1. False
In the South African Bantu, haemochromatosis caused by iron overload was previously comparatively common because of the fermentation of beer in iron utensils.

2. True
In both conditions excessive absorption of iron from the duodenum may occur, although haemosiderosis may also develop in haemolytic anaemias or following repeated blood transfusions. In hereditary haemochromatosis, the excessive absorption of intestinal iron leads to the accumulation of iron at the rate of 0.5–1.0 g/ annually. What

promotes the excessive absorption and the mechanism by which it is achieved is unknown.

3. False
When a systemic overload of iron occurs as in haemosiderosis, the pigment accumulates in the macrophages of the liver, bone marrow, spleen and lymph nodes and only later, as the load increases, in the parenchymal cells throughout the body. In haemochromatosis, iron is principally deposited in the parenchymal cells from the beginning leading to toxic effects in the affected cells, notably the liver, islet cells of the pancreas and the myocardium.

4. True
In hereditary haemochromatosis, because iron is toxic to the liver cells both micronodular cirrhosis and hepatocellular carcinoma may develop, either of which may be the ultimate cause of death.

5. False
The plasma transferrin is normal in quantity and not qualitatively abnormal in either condition.

SECTION 12. DISEASES OF THE LIVER AND GALL BLADDER

12.1 Obstruction of the common bile duct is associated with the following biochemical abnormalities:
1. a greater increase in the serum concentration of bilirubin diglucuronide than bilirubin monoglucuronide
2. an increase in the serum concentration of unconjugated bilirubin
3. a decrease in the faecal stercobilinogen content
4. an increase in faecal fat
5. an increase in urinary urobilinogen

1. False
The concentration of bilirubin monoglucuronide is increased relative to that of diglucuronide because biliary tract obstruction is associated with an impairment of conjugation as well as the more obvious obstructive element.

2. False
The serum concentration of conjugated bilirubin rises. Conjugated pigment is attached to serum protein, mainly albumin.

3. True
The stercobilinogen content of the faeces is dependent upon the amount of bilirubin excreted into the bowel. This is then converted to stercobilinogen by the intestinal flora.

4. True
The fat content of the faeces increases because in the absence of bile salts in the bowel fat absorption is diminished.

5. False
The urinary urobilinogen must decrease because it is derived from the stercobilinogen absorbed from the gastrointestinal tract some of which is excreted by the kidneys.

12.2 Haemolytic jaundice is associated with:
1. an increase in the concentration of bilirubin diglucuronide in the bile
2. the presence of bilirubin in the urine
3. an increase in the serum alkaline phosphatase
4. a decrease in unconjugated bilirubin in the serum
5. an increase in urobilinogen in the urine

1. True
Increased amounts of unconjugated bilirubin are presented to the liver cell. Because the liver cells are normal, conjugation proceeds normally and increased quantities of the diglucuronide appear in the bile.

2. False
Unconjugated bilirubin is insoluble in water unlike the conjugated forms and, therefore, does not appear in the urine in haemolytic anaemia, hence the term, acholuric jaundice.

3. False
The serum alkaline phosphatase concentration increases in obstructive and hepatocellular jaundice. Its concentration does not rise in haemolytic jaundice unless haemolysis has been associated with the formation of pigment stones which have then caused obstruction of the common bile duct.

4. False
In haemolytic disease, an increase in bilirubin occurs, principally of the unconjugated fraction. The total bilirubin rarely exceeds 5 mg/dl (85 μmol/l) because the rate of excretion increases as the total bilirubin rises and a plateau is quickly reached. Greater values suggest concomitant hepatic parenchymal disease.

5. True
Because increased quantities of conjugated bilirubin are being excreted into the gastrointestinal tract greater quantities of stercobilininogen are formed, absorbed and then excreted by the kidney as urobilinogen which is then converted to urobilin.

12.3 The common causes of cirrhosis of the liver in Great Britain are:
1. alcohol
2. drugs such as halothane and paracetamol
3. hepatitis B
4. haemochromatosis
5. primary biliary cirrhosis

1. True
In Great Britain as in the USA, alcohol abuse is the commonest cause of cirrhosis of the liver affecting in the U.K. about 1:10 chronic alcoholics. Whilst it is known that alcohol abuse produces a fatty liver, this is a reversible condition until fibrosis develops. Once this latter change occurs the condition becomes irreversible, ending in cirrhosis in which nodules of liver cells are encircled by fibrous tissue. Why some alcoholics develop cirrhosis and others remain immune is as yet unsolved. However, it is clearly established that the frequency of cirrhosis increases with the duration of abuse and the greater the quantity of alcohol consumed.

2. False
Halothane may produce a hepatitis indistinguishable from viral hepatitis; this is not however followed by cirrhosis. Likewise paracetamol, a commonly used analgesic, in doses in excess of 10 g may cause hepatic necrosis, the cause of which is attributed to a toxic metabolite which is normally detoxified by glutathione when the drug is given in normal dosage.

3. True
Hepatitis B, is caused by a member of the hepadoravirus family. It may cause acute hepatitis, a chronic non-progressive hepatitis, a fulminant hepatitis associated with massive liver necrosis, an asymptomatic carrier state with or without progressive disease and lastly a progressive chronic disease ending in cirrhosis. The latter situation arises in over one third of all patients suffering from chronic hepatitis. The cause of the damage to the liver cells is probably due to an immunological mechanism mediated via cytotoxic T cells, direct action of the virus itself appearing unlikely since no injury to hepatocytes is found in 'healthy' asymptomatic carriers.

4. False
Although haemochromatosis causes cirrhosis, it is a relatively rare cause in Britain.

5. False
Primary biliary cirrhosis eventually causes cirrhosis and liver failure but it is a rare condition. Primarily a disease of middle-aged women, the characteristic histological feature is one of a non-suppurative, granulomatous destruction of the medium sized hepatic ducts, cirrhosis developing only late in the course of the disease.
A prominent feature of PBC, is the appearance of anti-mitochondrial autoantibodies. The disease may be associated with other autoimmune diseases including Sjörgen's syndrome, scleroderma, Hashimoto's disease and rheumatoid arthritis, all conditions associated with an immunological derangement.

12.4 In liver failure the following biochemical abnormalities may be found:
1. a decrease in the plasma albumin concentration

2. an increase in the plasma globulin
3. an increase in the blood ammonium concentration
4. a rise in the blood urea
5. impaired glucose tolerance

1. True

The plasma albumin concentration usually falls in chronic liver disease, the majority of patients with cirrhosis having low albumin synthesis rates and small albumin pools.

2. True

The plasma globulin level is frequently increased in patients with cirrhosis because bacterial antigens derived from the gut may have access to the systemic circulation especially if a porta-caval shunt has been performed. In patients with autoimmune liver disease as part of the primary disease process serum autoantibodies will be present.

3. True

Ammonium is produced by the deamination of aminoacids and other nitrogenous substances in muscle, brain, kidney and the colon and cannot be converted to urea by the failing liver.

4. False

The blood urea does not rise unless there is associated renal failure because the ammonium cannot be converted into urea (see above).

5. True

Glucose tolerance is impaired in patients with acute hepatitis and reverts to normal with their clinical recovery. In fulminating hepatic failure the initial changes are similar and hypoglycaemia may supervene.

12.5 A diminution in the bile salt pool and hence a diminished concentration of bile salts in the bile occurs:
1. in jejunal diverticulosis
2. in diseases affecting the terminal ileum such as Crohn's disease
3. due to the eating of refined carbohydrates
4. in ulcerative colitis
5. in congenital deficiency of cholesterol 7α-hydroxylase

1. False

Bile salt depletion does not occur in jejunal diverticulosis because the absorption of bile salts occurs in the terminal ileum.

2. True

Bile salts are absorbed in the terminal ileum. Reabsorption is essential to preserve the enterohepatic circulation of the bile salts. If the terminal ileum is destroyed by disease or it is resected a diminished bile salt pool inevitably occurs. Because an adequate concentration of bile salts is required to hold the cholesterol in micelles any condition lowering the concentration of bile salts leads to an increased incidence of cholesterol gall stones.

3. True
There is some animal evidence that an acquired deficiency of the enzyme, cholesterol 7α-hydroxylase, follows the eating of refined carbohydrate. Deficiency of this enzyme causes a reduction in bile salt formation.

4. False
The diarrhoea associated with ulcerative colitis has no effect on the bile salt pool since the absorption of bile salts has already taken place in the terminal ileum.

5. True
A congenital deficiency of this enzyme leads to failure of bile salt synthesis.

12.6 Excessive cholesterol is excreted by the hepatocytes:
  1. when the diet contains excessive amounts of polyunsaturated fatty acids.
  2. in response to excessive secretion of testosterone
  3. when an individual is excessively obese
  4. when anticoagulants are administered in large doses
  5. when caloric intake is diminished

1. True
Both a diet containing an excess of polyunsaturated fatty acids and the administration of drugs such as Clofibrate increase the output of cholesterol.

2. False
Oestrogens increase cholesterol excretion. This is believed to be one of the causes of the greater incidence of 'metabolic stones' (cholesterol stones), in women.

3. True
Excessive obesity, probably because of the increase of body fat, causes an increase in the synthesis and excretion of cholesterol by the liver cells.

4. False
Anticoagulants have no effect on cholesterol metabolism.

5. False
A short-term increase in calorie intake may be associated with an increase in cholesterol excretion.

12.7 The main constituents of gall stones are:
  1. calcium sulphate
  2. cholesterol
  3. calcium palmitate

4. calcium bilirubinate
5. amorphous materials

1. False
No calcium sulphate is excreted in the bile. One third of the crystalline matter in stones found in Great Britain is calcium carbonate.

2. True
In developed countries, 80% of all gall stones are classified as cholesterol stones, containing 50% of crystalline cholesterol monohydrate. Cholesterol is rendered soluble in bile by aggregation with water soluble bile salts and water-insoluble lecithins, both of which act as detergents. If the cholesterol concentration exceeds the solubilising capacity of bile, i.e. the bile becomes supersaturated, the cholesterol is precipitated as solid cholesterol monohydrate. For a cholesterol stone to form, the cholesterol crystals must remain long enough in the gall bladder to aggregate into stones. Thus stasis is a potent factor in cholesterol stone formation, a common event during pregnancy, hence the prevalence of gall stones in the female.

3. True
Calcium palmitate is one of the lesser components of gall stones especially found in pigment stones.

4. True
Calcium bilirubinate is the major pigment found in pigment stones.

5. True
The amorphous material found in pigment stones is important because 90% of such stones are composed of this material which is chiefly a mucin glycoprotein.

12.8 Gall stones are associated with the following diseases:
1. viral hepatitis
2. cirrhosis of the liver
3. hereditary spherocytosis
4. obesity
5. raised serum triglycerides

1. False
Liver damage associated with viral hepatitis causes no increase in the incidence of gall stones.

2. False
Cirrhosis, although associated in the end stage with severe liver damage, does not increase the incidence of gall stones.

3. True
Hereditary spherocytosis is a condition characterized by an intrinsic defect in the red cell membrane which renders the red cell spheroidal in shape and less easily deformable. The abnormal red cells are trapped in the spleen and destroyed there, liberating haemoglobin

which is eventually excreted as excessive bilirubin leading to the formation of pigment stones in the gall bladder.

4. True
In one study of the incidence of gall stones in women below the age of fifty those with gall stones were 10 kilograms heavier than those without.

5. True
The incidence of gall stones is increased in conditions leading to a hyperlipidaemia causing an excess of serum triglycerides but not hypercholesterolaemia.

12.9 Severe liver failure is associated with:
1. mucosal bleeding
2. encephalopathy
3. bronchopneumonia
4. venous thrombosis
5. decreased resistance to infection

1. True
Mucosal bleeding from the upper gastrointestinal tract is relatively common and accounts for death in approximately 20% of all cases of advanced liver failure. Bleeding occurs from mucosal erosions and can be prevented by the administration of H_2 receptor antagonists.

2. True
The precise cause of hepatic encephalopathy is unknown. To develop the disorder two underlying situations must be present; (1) the shunting of blood away from the liver as occurs spontaneously in cirrhosis when portosystemic connections develop, or as a result of surgical interference following portocaval anastomosis and (2) severe loss of hepatocyte function. Despite the severe physiological effects which include confusion, coma and the 'flapping' tremor, the pathological changes in the brain itself are not marked and include only oedema and an astrocyte response.

3. True
Pulmonary complications in the form of bronchopneumonia are very common in severe liver failure due to the depression of the respiratory centre and a decreased resistance to infection.

4. False
Thrombosis is rare in severe liver disease because the synthesis of Factors II, V, VII, IX and X is impaired. In addition plasminogen activators may accumulate in the blood because the liver cannot metabolize them, with the result that a secondary fibrinolytic state develops.

5. True
The susceptibility to infection is increased in severe liver disease because the circulating toxins depress polymorphonuclear leucocyte activity and complement deficiency impairs bacterial opsonisation.

12.10 The following biochemical disturbances occur in fulminating hepatic failure:
1. metabolic acidosis
2. prolongation of the prothrombin time
3. hyperglycaemia
4. hyperbilirubinaemia
5. low serum albumin

1. True
A metabolic acidosis develops and reflects the profound tissue anoxia; its severity is an indicator of the prognosis.

2. True
The prothrombin time is prolonged because Factors I, II, V, VII and X are synthesized in the liver. When their concentration falls below 30% of their normal value, the prothrombin time increases and is a test of considerable prognostic significance.

3. False
Hyperglycaemia does not occur. Normally fulminating hepatic failure is accompanied by an increase in circulating insulin, impaired gluconeogenesis and an inability to mobilise the glycogen stores, thus producing a hypoglycaemic state.

4. True
The bilirubin always rises, reflecting the degree of jaundice.

5. False
The plasma albumin level remains normal unless the course of the disease is prolonged.

12.11 The following coagulation factors are generated in the liver:
1. Factor II
2. Factor IV
3. Factor VI
4. Factor XI
5. Factor X

The liver generates coagulation Factors II, V, VII, IX and X and all except Factor V are vitamin K dependent. Deficiencies of these factors together with disturbances in fibrinogen metabolism and thrombocytopenia account for the bleeding diathesis that accompanies both acute and chronic liver disease.

The correct answer to this question is, therefore,
1. True
2. False
3. False
4. True
5. True

SECTION 13. CARCINOGENESIS

13.1 A hereditary predisposition to the development of tumours occurs in the following sites:
1. Retina
2. Colon
3. Uterus
4. Skin
5. Stomach

1. True
Between 6–10% of retinoblastomas are familiar when the tumour is nearly always bilateral, whereas in sporadic cases the tumour is more commonly unilateral. In the familial type, such patients are also at risk of developing osteosarcoma and soft tissue tumours. In the familial disease a mutant Rb gene is present, localized on chromosome Bq14, but in order to develop a tumour the intact copy of the gene must be lost in the retinoblasts through some form of somatic mutation.

2. True
The classic disorder of the colon which predisposes to the eventual development of malignancy in 100% of those affected is familial polyposis. This is transmitted in an autosomal dominant fashion. Typically the colon becomes carpeted at an early age by adenomata, the majority of which are of the tubular variety although some may have villous characteristics. The gene associated with FP has been mapped at chromosome 5q21.

3. False
There is no hereditary predisposition to endometrial cancer. The most significant factor in the development of endometrial cancer is prolonged oestrogen stimulation and endometrial hyperplasia. The importance of endometrial hyperplasia is borne out by the increased risk of endometrial cancer in females with oestrogen secreting tumours of the ovary, the increased risk in women receiving hormone replacement therapy and the decreased incidence of this disease in women castrated in early life or suffering from ovarian agenesis.

4. True
Both malignant melanoma and basal cell carcinomata have been shown in some cases to be due to an hereditary predisposition. In the case of MM, genetic analysis has shown that the trait is inherited as an autosomal dominant, possibly involving a gene in the short arm of chromosome 1, near the Rh locus. In these cases the melanoma develops from a dysplastic naevus. In the case of inherited basal cell tumours, the tumours develop early in life and are commonly associated with abnormalities of bone, the nervous system, eyes and the reproductive organs.

5. False
Carcinoma of the stomach shows no hereditary predisposition,

although this tumour is more common in individuals with blood group A and there is an increased incidence in some racial groups, e.g. the Japanese.

13.2 Recognised precancerous conditions include:
1. the intestinal polyps of the small bowel occurring in the Peutz–Jegher syndrome
2. the colonic polyps of familial polyposis
3. xeroderma pigmentosum
4. Bowen's disease
5. molluscum sebaceum

1. False
The Peutz–Jeghers syndrome is a rare autosomal dominant condition in which multiple hamartomatous polyps develop throughout the gastrointestinal tract in association with hyperpigmentation around the lips, on the oral mucosa, genitalia and the palmar surface of the hands. Although the polyps themselves have no malignant potential, individuals suffering from this condition have an increased risk of developing carcinoma of the breast and lung.

2. True
By definition familial polyposis is a condition in which a minimum of 100 polyps develop in the colon, although in the majority of cases many thousands may be present. The polyps appear in the second and third decades of life and within some 10–15 years become overtly malignant.

3. True
Xeroderma pigmentosa is a condition in which affected individuals are extremely photosensitive and in which there is an inherited inability to repair damage to DNA following exposure to ultraviolet light which causes the formation of pyrimidine dimers. The inability to repair these dimers results in an increased frequency of mutations leading to the early development of malignancy.

4. True
Bowen's disease affects the genital regions in both males and females. Grossly the condition appears as a solitary grey-white plaque associated with ulceration. Histologically the epidermis shows proliferation and numerous mitoses. The cells are markedly dysplastic but the dermal–epidermal boundary is sharply delineated by an intact basement membrane. In approximately 10–30% of sufferers however, over a period of many years the lesion becomes transformed into a typical squamous carcinoma.

5. False
This tumour-like lesion occurs predominantly on the face and has a natural history of approximately six months. A nodule appears which grows rapidly for about eight weeks during which time the histological picture resembles that of a squamous carcinoma. After this the lesion

stabilises and the exuberant epithelium which has formed slowly keratinises. This is then discharged and the lesion heals.

13.3 The following pathological conditions can be regarded as precancerous:
1. osteitis deformans
2. leukoplakia
3. fibroadenosis of the breast
4. duodenal ulceration
5. cervical erosions

1. True
Osteitis deformans also known as Paget's disease is a chronic bone dystrophy of unknown aetiology. Commonly it is polyostotic affecting the pelvis, spine and skull, but in about 15% of cases it is monostotic when it usually affects the tibia, ilium, femur or a single vertebral body. Histologically it is a disease marked by phases of bone resorption followed by bone formation. The net effect is an increase in bone mass which has a distorted architectural appearance. Although not considered a metabolic disorder, the serum alkaline phosphatase is raised and the urinary excretion of hydroxyproline is increased. Between 5–10% of patients affected by polyostotic disease develop osteosarcoma.

2. True
Leukoplakia is a clinical term indicating the presence of white patches in a squamous epithelial mucous membrane. The condition affects the oral cavity and the vulva. In the mouth the condition is believed to be precipitated by chronic irritation. The whiteness of the affected epithelial surface is due to thickening of the epithelium and prolongation of the rete pegs. The papillae contain a chronic inflammatory infiltrate. As time passes the whiteness of the epithelium is converted to reddening due to a loss of cellular thickness and finally a carcinoma *in situ* develops leading eventually to invasive squamous carcinoma. The incidence of overt malignancy in leukoplakia is of the order of 5%. The onset of malignancy is clinically recognisable by the development of warty thickening within the plaques.

3. False
Fibroadenosis of the breast, previously known as chronic mastitis and now as generalized cystic mastopathy, does not predispose to neoplastic change unless it is accompanied by marked epithelial hyperplasia. The latter is one of the four possible pathological changes seen in the breast, the others being fibrosis, cyst formation and adenosis. Adenosis indicates the formation of new breast lobules and/or the enlargement of pre-existing one. The epithelial hyperplasia if referred to as epitheliosis, a term coined by Dawson to indicate hyperplasia of the ductal and acinar epithelium. It is only when this change is marked that the condition can be regarded as precancerous.

4. False
Neoplastic changes do not appear to supervene in duodenal ulceration.

5. False
The term cervical erosion is applied to the appearance of a red area around the external os spreading onto the exocervix. Histological examination shows that the normal opaque squamous epithelium has been replaced by transparent columnar epithelium. Should the replacement involve the cervical glands an appearance may be produced which is sometimes mistakenly interpreted as early invasive carcinomatous change.

13.4 The following are carcinogenic:
1. infra-red radiation
2. ultra-violet radiation
3. house dust
4. soot
5. moulds

1. False
Long wave infra-red irradiation is not associated with tumour development.

2. True
The ultraviolet portion of the solar spectrum is divisible into wavelengths. Of these, the middle band with a wave length of 280–320 nm is believed to be the cause of skin cancers and melanomata. The carcinogenic effect is believed to be due to the formation of pyrimidine dimers in DNA which, when unrepaired, lead to larger transcriptional errors and in some cases malignancy. The degree of risk from UVR not only depends on its wavelength but also on the intensity of exposure and the quantity of light absorbing melanin in the skin. Thus UVR is a more potent carcinogen in fair skinned people.

3. False
There are no carcinogens in normal house dust. This should be compared to some industrial occupations, e.g. workers in asbestos factories, in which dust may play an important role in the development of malignant disease. A condition associated with house dust is allergy, causing hay fever and bronchial asthma, chiefly due to antigens from the house dust mite, *Dermatophagoides pteronyssinus*.

4. True
Soot is a carcinogenic agent because of its contained coal tar products including 3.4 benzpyrene. Cancer of the scrotum occurring in chimney sweeps was the first occupational cancer to be described by Percival Pott in 1775.

5. True
Aflatoxin is a carcinogen produced by *Aspergillus flavus*, a species of Aspergillus found on the surface of peanuts. It is believed to be a major cause of hepatocellular cancer in the black population of Africa.

13.5 The following chemicals are indirect-acting carcinogens, i.e. require metabolic conversion to become carcinogenic:
1. 1, 2, 5, 6 dibenzanthrazine
2. cyclophosphamide
3. β-napthylamine
4. acetyl salicylic acid
5. 4-dimethylamino-azobenzene

1. False
Applied to the skin of mice this chemical acts to initiate cellular changes by causing permanent damage to the cellular DNA. When stimulated by a wide range of non-specific substances such as phenol, turpentine or croton oil in the area previously treated by an initiator a malignant tumour develops, the latter substances acting as promoters (or co-carcinogens). In the absence of a promoter carcinogenesis does not occur.

2. False
Cyclophosphamide is a weak direct acting carcinogen like other alkylating agents in this group. Because the alkylating agents exert their therapeutic effects as anticancer agents by damaging cellular DNA, it is this same action which renders them direct carcinogenic agents.

3. True
In the past β-napthylamine was responsible for the high incidence of bladder cancer in workers in the aniline dye and rubber industries. After absorption it is hydroxylated into an active carcinogen and then detoxified by conjugation with glucuronic acid. When excreted in the urine, the non-carcinogenic conjugate is split by the urinary enzyme gluronidase to release the active electrophilic reactant which is carcinogenic.

4. False
Aspirin is a potent cause of gastric erosions and thus gastric bleeding but so far no association has been found between it and tumour formation.

5. True
4-dimethylamino-azobenzene or butter yellow has been used for colouring foodstuffs. Fed to rats and mice it is a potent inducer of hepatic cancers.

13.6 The following occupations have been or remain associated with a high incidence of cancer:
1. coal mining

2. nickel workers
3. asbestos workers
4. beryllium workers
5. tobacco industry

1. False
Although there is a high incidence of pneumoconiosis, silicosis, tuberculosis and chronic bronchitis in coal miners, there is no evidence of an increased incidence of neoplasia directly related to this industry. Coal tar on the other hand contains potent carcinogens.

2. True
A higher incidence of bronchial cancer and cancer of the nasal sinuses occurs in workers in contact with nickel or chrome. This is related to the inhalation of dust containing these materials.

3. True
Workers who inhale asbestos have a higher than normal incidence of all types of cancer of the lung. The inhalation of blue asbestos is particularly associated with the development of mesotheliomas. Asbestos exists in two distinct geometric forms, the serpentine chrysolite chemical which is composed of curly flexible fibres and the amphibole type composed of straight, stiff brittle fibres. The amphiboles include crocidolite and various other forms and this is the type which is particularly associated with the development of mesothelioma, although both types promote severe pulmonary interstitial fibrosis.

4. False
Beryllium is used in combination with copper as an alloy in many industries because of its high tensile strength and its resistance to metal fatigue and corrosion. It is not associated with malignancy but causes a systemic disease predominantly affecting the lungs, causing a diffuse chronic non-caseating interstitial granulomatosis which may ultimately lead to death from cardio-pulmonary failure.

5. False
The preparation of tobacco and cigarettes does not hold any risk for industrial workers. The carcinogens in tobacco are coal tar products which form only when the tobacco is smoked. Nicotine is not carcinogenic.

13.7 The following infections are associated with the development of cancer:
1. clostridial infections
2. HBV infection
3. EBV infection
4. chlamydial infections
5. schistosomiasis

1. False
Clostridia are Gram-positive anaerobic spore bearing organisms and

are not known to have any neoplastic association. *Clostridium welchii, oedematiens* and *histolyticum* cause gas gangrene with *Cl. welchii* also causing severe food poisoning. *Clostidium tetani* causes tetanus and *Clostridium botulinus*, botulism, a severe and often fatal toxaemic disease resulting from the ingestion of contaminated food.

2. True

Hepatitis B virus infection, the cause of 'serum hepatitis' is associated in two ways with hepatocellular carcinoma of the liver:

(1) an acute infection may be followed by a persistent infection which may progress to chronic hepatitis followed by cirrhosis. In about 10% of patients so affected a hepatocellular carcinoma develops.

(2) in areas of the world in which the prevalence of HBV infection is high as in some parts of Africa, e.g. Mozambique, a high incidence of hepatocellular carcinoma occurs. In these cases the HBV infection begins in infancy folllowing a vertical transmission from the mother, this results in a carrier state in which there is a 200 fold increased risk of developing HCC in early adult life, not necessarily associated with pre-existing cirrhosis.

3. True

The Epstein–Barr virus, a member of the herpes family, has been implicated in four different types of human tumour, Burkitt's lymphoma, B-cell lymphoma in imunosuppressed individuals, particularly if they have been infected with the human immunosuppressed deficiency virus, some cases of Hodgkin's disease and nasopharyngeal carcinomata. EBV infects the epithelium of the nasopharynx and B lymphocytes. Burkitt's lymphoma is a neoplasm of B lymphocytes and is the most common childhood tumour in Central Africa and New Guinea.

4. False

The chlamydia are not associated with neoplastic disease, They are infectious agents about 300 nm in diameter which cause trachoma, ophthalmia neonatorum, lymphogranuloma venereum and psittacosis. They cannot be cultured on normal culture media and have to be grown in eggs or tissue culture.

5. True

The deposition of schistosome eggs in the wall of the bladder causes metaplasia of the bladder mucosa to occur from the normal transitional cell to a squamous cell epithelium. The great majority of bladder tumours developing in schistosomiasis are of squamous type, only about 30% being transitional cell carcinoma.

13.8 An increase in the frequency of malignant disease occurs in the following conditions:

1. following the long term administration of immunosuppressive agents
2. large bowel Crohn's disease

3. coeliac disease
4. ulcerative colitis
5. xeroderma pigmentosum

1. True
Following homotransplantation, long term immunosuppressive therapy is required. In such patients continued suppression of the immune system leads to the development of lymphomas, most commonly immunoblastic B-cell lymphomas. Other types of tumour are rarely encountered.

2. False
Malignant disease does not appear to follow long term granulomatous disease of the large bowel.

3. True
In coeliac disease, otherwise known as gluten sensitive enteropathy, there is a long term risk of T-cell lymphomas developing in the small bowel. The fundamental disorder is a sensitivity to gluten which contains the protein component of wheat known as gliadin. Large numbers of B cells sensitised to gliadin appear in the small bowel mucosa and biopsy shows marked atrophy and blunting of the villi, but increased mitotic activity in the crypts.

4. True
Chronic ulcerative colitis is followed by an increase in large bowel malignancy. All recorded series show that the incidence of malignancy in this disease increases with the length of the clinical history and the severity of the disease.

5. True
Xeroderma pigmentosum is a classical premalignant condition. Sufferers from this inherited disease rapidly develop skin cancer after exposure to ultra violet light.

13.9 An enhancement of tumour growth or an increased incidence of tumour formation may occur:
1. following the long term administration of immunosuppressive drugs
2. following immunological enhancement
3. due to the release of soluble antigens by the tumour cells
4. due to an alteration of T-cell function
5. due to the excessive production or release of lysosomal enzymes

1. True
An increase in the incidence on non-Hodgkin's lymphoma has been reported in patients undergoing long term immunosuppressive treatment with drugs such as azathioprine. This drug is commonly used following renal transplantation or for the treatment of autoimmune diseases such as systemic lupus erythematosus.

2. True
Immunological enhancement of tumour growth develops because of the production of 'blocking' antibody. This protects the tumour antigens from any cell-mediated immune response which the presence of the tumour provokes. In an experimental animal immunological enhancement of a transplantable tumour can be provoked by the prior immunization of the recipient with a dead tumour extract before the injection of live tumour cells.

3. True
Tumours may shed soluble tumour specific transplantation antigens (TSTA) into the circulation which then react with the antigen reactive sites on effector T cells thus reducing the severity of the cell-mediated immune response mounted to effect destruction of the tumour. This is one of the causes of a tumour 'sneaking through' a powerful immune response.

4. True
T lymphocytes may exert a suppressor as well as an effector action in the body's immune response mounted against a tumour. The suppressor T lymphocytes form a distinct sub-population differing from the effector cells and distinguished by their different surface (Ly) antigens. A balance between suppressor and effector lymphocytes forms the regulatory basis of the immune response.

5. False
Lysosomal enzymes, chiefly found in the macrophages, are important in degrading antigen prior to its presentation to the lymphocytes. These enzymes are mainly hydrolytic and proteolytic and thus are effective, following the activation of the macrophages by lymphokine, in destroying tumour cells and microorganisms which have undergone phagocytosis.

13.10 The following are specific markers for certain specific types of malignancy:
1. 5-HIAA
2. α-fetoprotein
3. Bence–Jones protein
4. chorionic gonadotrophin
5. carcinoembryonic antigen

1. True
5-HIAA is a specific marker for carcinoid tumours of the gastrointestinal tract, 5-hydroxyindoleacetic acid is the inactive metabolite of 5-hydroxytryptamine. Increased levels occur in the blood in patients suffering from carcinoid tumours of the gastrointestinal tract because 5HT, if secreted by the tumour, is degraded in the liver.

2. False
α-fetoprotein is a glycoprotein normally synthesized in early fetal life

by the yolk sac, fetal liver and gastrointestinal tract. Abnormal levels
are particularly found in adult life in some 60–70% of patients
suffering from hepatocellular carcinoma of the liver, embryonal
carcinomas and yolk sac tumours of the testes. However, the
presence of this substance is not conclusive evidence of malignancy
since elevated levels may occur in cirrhosis, massive liver necrosis
and fetal neural abnormalities.

3. True
Bence–Jones proteins are free light chains of the immunoglobulin
molecules that are present in the urine in patients suffering from
multiple myeloma. They have α or λ antigenic determinants. These
proteins precipitate on heating the urine to 80°C but return into
solution at higher temperatures.

4. True
Large amounts of chorionic gonadothrophin are produced in normal
pregnancy and following the development of hydatidiform moles or
choriocarcinoma. In the latter, therefore, urine pregnancy tests are
strongly positive.

5. False
CEA is normally produced in the embryonic tissue of the gut,
pancreas and the liver. It is a complex glycoprotein elaborated by
many different neoplasms. Thus it is present in some 60–90% of
patients suffering from carcinoma of the colon, 50–80% suffering
from pancreatic neoplasms and 50% suffering from gastric or
mammary cancer. It may also rise in non-neoplastic conditions such
as Crohn's disease and ulcerative colitis and hepatitis. However in
colonic carcinoma, the level correlates with the tumour load and an
elevated level following treatment is indicative of residual disease.

13.11 The incidence of tumours is increased in:
1. sarcoidosis
2. Wiskott–Aldrich syndrome
3. ataxia telangiectasis
4. patients treated over long periods with corticosteroids
5. patients receiving azathioprine

1. False
Despite the depression of certain parameters of T-lymphocyte
function which occurs in sarcoidosis there is no evidence of any
increase in the incidence of malignancy in this disease.

2. True
The Wiskott–Aldrich syndrome is a sex linked recessive disease
which causes the affected children to suffer from atopic eczema,
thrombocytopenia and an increased susceptibility to infection.
Although the thymus is morphologically normal, there is a
progressive secondary depletion of T lymphocytes in the peripheral
blood and the paracortical areas of the lymph nodes. The serum

contains increased amounts of IgA and IgE, normal of IgG but decreased amounts of IgM. Eventually failure of T-lymphocyte function is followed by an increased incidence of lymphomas.

3. True
Ataxia telangiectasis is an autosomal recessive condition in which the thymus is hypoplastic. Delayed hypersensitivity reactions are depressed and plasma concentrations of IgA and IgG fall. A considerable number of patients develop malignant lymphomas or lymphatic leukaemia. The disease usually presents in infancy with cerebellar ataxia due to the associated atrophy of the cerebellar cortex and demyelination of the cerebellar peduncles.

4. False
There is no evidence that prolonged treatment with corticosteroids predisposes to tumour development.

5. True
In any patient receiving immunosuppressive drugs over long periods there is an increased incidence of lymphophomas.

SECTION 14. TUMOURS

14.1 A tumour may be defined as:
1. an abnormal mass of tissue
2. a growth of tissue which exceeds and is uncoordinated with that of normal tissues
3. a growth of tissue which is limited and coordinated with that of the rest of the body
4. an abnormal increase in the cells of a tissue
5. a malformation in which the various tissues of the part are present in improper proportions or distribution

1. True
This is the opening phrase of the definition of a tumour as proposed by the late Professor R. A. Willis.

2. True
This is the second part of the definition of a tumour as constructed by Willis. It is followed by a third part, i.e. the growth of the tumour persists in the same excessive manner after cessation of the stimulus or stimuli which evoked the change.

3. False
A tissue, the growth of which is limited and coordinated with that of the rest of the body, is a malformation. A classic example is the cutaneous angioma, otherwise known as the 'port-wine stain' which grows only with the growth of the rest of the body and does not extend to involve a greater and greater territory of tissue.

4. False
This is the simple definition of hyperplasia. Hyperplasia usually occurs as:
  (a) A compensatory response to loss of tissue of the same kind
  (b) An increased functional demand which cannot be satisfied by the tissue already present
  (c) Disturbed hormonal control of the activity of the tissue.

5. False
This is the definition of a hamartoma.

14.2 Broder's classification of tumours attempted to classify tumours according to:
1. their origin
2. the degree of differentiation of a tumour
3. the degree of stromal response
4. the degree of lymphocytic infiltration of the tumour
5. the number of mitoses found in a given area of the tumour

1. False
Broder worked mainly with tumours of squamous epithelium.

2. True
This was the fundamental basis of Broder's classification. He recognised four grades of malignancy according to the degree of differentiation of the tumour. Grade 1, when more than 75% of the tumour cells were differentiated; Grade 4, when less than 25% of the tumour cells were differentiated with intermediate values in grades 2 and 3. This classification has been abandoned for many reasons:
  (a) It is time consuming and, therefore, expensive
  (b) Different parts of a tumour may show entirely different histological characteristics
  (c) The results did not always correspond to the prognosis which is what Broder sought to establish. Thus a Grade 1 tumour of the skin has excellent prognosis whereas a Grade 1 bronchial carcinoma has a poor prognosis.

3. False
Stromal response, particularly of breast tumours, has been shown to influence prognosis but was not taken into account by Broder who was chiefly concerned with skin cancer.

4. False
Lymphocytic infiltration was not considered in Broder's classification although some importance is now attributed to this aspect. The degree of lymphocytic infiltration is regarded by many pathologists as an indication of the body's immunological response to the tumour.

5. True
The number of mitoses indicates a greater degree of malignancy. Various modifications of Broder's original classification have been

proposed one of which, applied by Greenhough to breast tumours, took into account three features of these glandular carcinomata:
(a) Tubule formation
(b) The regularity in size, shape and staining of the nuclei of the tumour cells
(c) Number of mitoses.

14.3 Neoplastic disease may be associated with the following conditions:
1. dermatomyositis
2. acanthosis nigricans
3. necrobiosis lipoidica
4. thrombophlebitis migrans
5. polyarteritis nodosa

1. True
Approximately 20% of patients suffering from dermatomyositis have an underlying malignant condition. Dermatomyositis is an inflammatory lesion of muscle in which a mononuclear infiltrate occurs between the muscle bundles which themselves show mild degrees of degeneration and a loss of the normal transverse striations. The cutaneous lesions consist of erythematous patches with slight oedema. The classic rash takes the form of a lilac or heliotrope discolouration of the upper eyelids accompanied by periorbital oedema. Clinically, there is muscle weakness.

2. True
Acanthosis nigricans is characterized by grey-black patches of verrucous hyperkeratosis. It is associated with visceral malignancy and occasionally with Hodgkin's disease or osteogenic sarcoma.

3. False
Necrobiosis lipoidica is not associated with neoplasia. It is a condition in which yellowish demarcated lesions develop on the shins, the centre of which become atrophic, breaking down to form ulcers. Histologically the lesions may be necrobiotic and granulomatous. Diabetes is the underlying disease in approximately two thirds of affected individuals.

4. True
Thrombophlebitis migrans is chiefly associated with tumours of the pancreas, lung, stomach and female genital tract. Clinically, repeated attacks of segmental thrombosis occurs in both the superficial and the deep veins, attacks which heal spontaneously.

5. False
Polyarteritis nodosa is not associated with malignant disease but with hypersensitivity to a number of drugs including the sulphonamides and the anti-inflammatory agents such as phenylbutazone. It also

occurs in HBV infections. The underlying cause is immune complex disease resulting in a necrotising arteritis affecting both deep and superficial vessels accompanied by a polymorphonuclear leucocyte infiltration around the vessels.

14.4 General phenomena associated with neoplasia may include:
1. fever
2. cachexia
3. thrombotic episodes
4. polycythaemia
5. dermatomyositis

1. True
Fever, unassociated with infection, is particularly associated with the following tumours:
  (a) Nephroblastoma
  (b) Carcinoma of the renal tubules (hypernephroma)
  (c) Lymphomata.
The cause of such pyrexia remains uncertain although it must be due to pyrogens formed by the breakdown products of the tumour.

2. True
Cachexia is one of the common manifestations of widespread and terminal malignancy. The cause may be difficult to identify but in gastrointestinal tumours loss of appetite, bleeding and sepsis play a part.

3. True
The classic thrombotic episode associated with neoplasia is that described by Trousseau in 1865, of recurrent superficial and deep venous thrombosis which undergo spontaneous remission; thrombophlebitis migrans. Rarely, a non-bacterial thrombotic endocarditis occurs in widespread malignant disease and even rarer is disseminated intravascular coagulation.

4. True
Polycythaemia does not normally complicate neoplasia, indeed the reverse is usually the case due either to blood loss, invasion of the red marrow or as yet unidentified causes. One exception is renal carcinoma which, by producing excessive erythropoietin, leads to a polycythaemia.

5. True
Dermatomyositis is a disorder which affects the skin, muscles and blood vessels. A coagulative necrosis occurs together with a small round cell infiltration around the smaller arteries. Approximately 30% of all patients suffering from dermatomyositis between 50 and 70 years of age are found to be suffering from disseminated malignant disease usually arising from the gastrointestinal tract and less frequently the bladder and bronchus.

14.5 The following tumours may secrete hormones:
1. carcinoid tumours
2. choriocarcinoma
3. benign teratoma of the ovary
4. monodermal teratoma of the ovary
5. seminoma

1. True
Carcinoid tumours occur primarily in the gastrointestinal tract, most commonly in the ileum but they can in fact arise anywhere along the whole length of the gut and also in the bronchial tree, pancreas, biliary tree and ovary. The carcinoid syndrome, due to the secretion of 5HT (serotonin) arises in about 1% of all patients who develop a carcinoid whatever the primary site and in 20% of those in whom a gastrointestinal tumour develops associated with hepatic metastases. The importance of liver metastases is that serotonin is normally metabolized by the liver to an inactive end product 5-HIAA (5-hydroxyindole acetic acid). The release of 5HT causes intermittent flushing of the face, an increase in intestinal motility leading to diarrhoea and lesions on the pulmonary or tricuspid valves causing right sided heart failure.

2. True
Choriocarcinomas produce excessive quantities of chorionic gonadotrophin with the result that severe uterine bleeding occurs. Approximately 50% follow the development of a hydatidiform mole whilst 25% develop following perfectly normal pregnancies.

3. False
Benign teratoma of the ovary are usually cystic forming the so-called dermoid cyst of the ovary. They give rise to no hormonal secretions.

4. True
Monodermal or specialised teratomas are a rare group of ovarian tumours the most common of which are struma ovarii and carcinoid. Struma ovarii are composed of mature thyroid cells and may cause hyperthyroidism and carcinoid tumours of the ovary may, when large, give rise to the carcinoid syndrome.

5. True
The majority of seminomas of the testes do not secrete hormones but in approximately 10%, synctial giant cells that resemble the syncytiotrophoblasts of the placenta are present. These cells secrete HGH (human gonadothrophic hormone) the serum level of which is raised.

14.6 Exfoliative cytology is useful for the diagnosis of:
1. meningioma
2. bronchial cancer
3. multiple myeloma

4. cervical cancer
5. vesical cancer

1. False
The examination of cerebro-spinal fluid for exfoliated cells has not been shown to be particularly useful in the diagnosis of tumours of the CNS. Meningiomas do not generally shed cells into the CSF.

2. True
Malignant cells can be demonstrated in the sputum, bronchial washings and if present, in a pleural effusion, in patients suffering from bronchial cancer.

3. False
Although malignant plasma cells may be demonstrated occasionally in the peripheral blood in patients with multiple myeloma, this cannot strictly be called exfoliative cytology. Malignant cells in this condition are usually sought in marrow specimens.

4. True
Vaginal and cervical smears are commonly used to eliminate or confirm a diagnosis of carcinoma of the cervix or uterus. The abnormal cells which are pleomorphic and hyperchromatic are demonstrated by the use of a 'Papanicolaou' smear. This technique may also identify carcinoma *in situ* and various forms of dysplasia.

5. True
Exfoliative cytology is used extensively for the exclusion or diagnosis of tumours of the bladder. It is also extensively used in the screening of asymptomatic individuals working in the aniline dye industry.

14.7 The findings of the following substances in excessive quantities in the blood may be due to the presence of a specific type of tumour:
1. noradrenaline
2. 5-hydroxytryptamine
3. carcinoembryonic antigen
4. prostaglandins
5. calcium

1. True
Excessive noradrenaline may indicate the presence of a phaeochromocytoma although this tumour also produces excessive quantities of adrenaline. The presenting symptoms of these tumours are determined by the relative concentration of the two hormones.

2. True
Excessive 5-hydroxytryptamine (serotonin) indicates the presence of a carcinoid tumour otherwise known as an argentaffinoma because the cytoplasm of the tumour cell can form deposits of silver from silver salts.

3. True
Carcinoembryonic antigen, one of the oncofetal antigens, is associated with gastrointestinal tumours. An estimation of this marker is of little initial assistance in their diagnosis but it is of some value as an indicator of metastatic recurrence since above normal values suggest that hepatic metastases have developed.

4. False
Although prostaglandins are found in a variety of tissues such as the seminal vesicles, lung, iris and renal medulla no tumour has been described in which this group of compounds is produced in excessive quantities.

5. True
Hypercalcaemia may indicate the presence of a benign or malignant parathyroid tumour or more commonly the presence of extensive osseous metastases. The latter arise most commonly from primary tumours of the breast, thyroid, bronchus, kidney or prostate.

14.8 Neuroblastomas are most common in:
1. children
2. may differentiate into benign tumours
3. the adrenal medulla
4. the floor of the fourth ventricle
5. sympathetic ganglia

1. True
Neuroblastomas are one of the most common extracranial solid tumours of childhood accounting for some 20% of all deaths from malignant disease. In all, 90% occur below 5 years of age. The majority are sporadic but in about one quarter there is evidence of a hereditary disposition.

2. True
Although rare, neuroblastomas may differentiate into benign ganglioneuroma.

3. True
Almost one third of all neuroblastomas arise in the adrenal medulla. Arising in this site, they give rise to two distinct clinical syndromes, Pepper's syndrome associated with hepatomegaly and Hutchinson's syndrome associated with osseous metastases in the periorbital and orbital bones giving rise to periorbital bruising and possibly exophthalmos.

4. False
Rarely primary neuroblastomas do arise within the brain and are to be found in the cerebral hemispheres. The commonest intracranial tumour of nervous origin in childhood is the medulloblastoma which develops almost exclusively in the cerebellum. These latter tumours are highly malignant.

5. True

Neuroblastoma, otherwise known as sympatheticoblastoma may arise in the sympathetic ganglia. Regardless of the site of origin, there is a considerable degree of differentiation. Most are composed of small cells containing darkly staining nuclei and scant cytoplasm. A typical appearance is the arrangement of these cells in rosettes, the central spaces of which are filled with fibrillar extensions of the cells.

14.9 Hormone dependency may be exhibited by the following tumours:
1. malignant melanoma
2. prostatic carcinoma
3. follicular carcinoma of the thyroid
4. bronchial carcinoma
5. retinoblastoma

1. True

Although hormone therapy has no beneficial effect on malignant melanoma well documented reports do appear in the literature of such tumours regressing during pregnancy, presumably due to its hormonal effects.

2. True

The scientific basis of hormone dependency was first established by Charles Huggins of Chicago after the Second World War when he discovered that carcinoma of the prostate was affected by altering its hormonal environment. Later he discovered that oophorectomy and adrenalectomy had a beneficial effect on disseminated breast cancer. It is interesting to note, however, that Beatson and others in the early part of this century had observed that the former operation sometimes produced great, although temporary, improvement in advanced breast cancer.

3. True

The growth of both follicular and papillary tumours of the thyroid may be suppressed by the administration of thyroxine.

4. False

Bronchial carcinomata are not hormone dependent although they occasionally produce hormones, in particular ACTH. When this occurs Cushingoid features develop.

5. False

This is a tumour of infancy of which about 6% of cases are familial. There is no evidence of hormone dependency.

14.10 The commonest tumours of the central nervous system arise from:
1. the meninges
2. primary tumours elsewhere in the body

3. neuroglia
4. the blood vessels
5. nerve cells

1. False
Meningioma, developing from the arachnoid cells which lie in the deep surface of the dura, are only the third commonest tumour of the central nervous system.

2. True
Secondary metastatic deposits are the commonest single group of tumours of the central nervous system. The tumours which most commonly metastasize to the central nervous system arise from the breast, bronchus, skin, melanoma and the gastrointestinal tract.

3. True
Tumours of the neuroglia are known as glioma. The tumours of this group include astrocytomas, oligodendrogliomas and ependymomas. Approximately 80% of adult brain tumours are classified as fibrillary astrocytomas which most commonly arise in the cerebral hemispheres in late middle age.

4. False
True tumours of the blood vessels of the brain are rare. Harmartomatous malformations form about 2% of cerebral tumours.

5. False
Tumours of the central nervous system which arise from mature-looking neurons do occur but are rare. Usually such tumours are a mixture of both ganglion cells and glial cells forming tumours known as gangliogliomas. Pure gangliocytomas occur in the floor of the third ventricle, the hypothalamus and the temporal lobes. Their degree of malignancy is related to any glial content present in the tumour.

14.11 The 'doubling time' of a malignant tumour is affected by a number of factors including:
1. a decrease in cell cycle time
2. exfoliation
3. the percentage of cells in the resting phase
4. the oxygen content of the tumour cells environment
5. nuclear size

1. False
The cell cycle time of tumour cells is unrelated to the growth of a tumour because although tumour cells pass through the same cell cycle as normal cells, i.e. Go, G1, S, G2 and M, measurements suggest that the duration of these phases is for many tumours equal or longer than that of the normal cells from which the tumour is derived.

2. True
Exfoliation is a significant factor leading to the loss of tumour cells

capable of division. This feature is particularly important in tumours of the gastrointestinal tract and urothelium.

3. True
The percentage of cells in the resting phase certainly determines the 'doubling time' of a tumour. The number of cells not in the resting phase, the growth fraction, appears to be high in the early phase of tumour growth, but as the tumour grows in size, cells leave the replicative pool in increasing numbers returning to the Go and G1 phase. Different tumours have different growth fractions; thus some leukaemias and lymphomas have high fractions particularly when compared to more solid tumours. A further complication affecting the growth of a tumour is the heterogenous nature of the cell population; thus some clones of tumour cells may only be capable of four or five divisions before dying.

4. True
Tumour cells in culture can form nodules between 1–2 mm in diameter before requiring a blood supply. However in solid tumours, necrosis occurs when the tumour extends more than 1–2 mm beyond a tumour blood vessel, indicating that beyond this limit the oxygen and nutritional requirements of the tumour cell cannot be sustained.

5. False
Nuclear size bears no relationship to the time taken for the division of malignant cells.

14.12 The interphase is:
1. situated between the prophase and metaphase
2. a resting stage between cell division
3. associated with growth of a cell
4. accompanied by the accumulation of RNA
5. situated between the anaphase and the telophase

1. False
The prophase may be regarded as the beginning of cell division. During this phase the chromosomes become visible and during the metaphase the spindle is formed radiating from the centrioles situated at opposite poles of the cell.

2. True
During the interphase chromosomes cannot be detected within the nucleus as discrete structures by a light microscope.

3. True
The interphase is associated with the accumulation of ribonucleic acid in the cell.

4. True

5. False
The interphase follows the telophase during which the chromosomes elongate and disappear as the new nuclear membrane forms and the spindle disappears.

14.13 The embryonic tumours of infancy include:
1. nephroblastoma
2. osteogenic sarcoma (osteosarcoma)
3. medulloblastoma
4. cholangiocarcinoma
5. lympho-epithelioma

1. True
This renal neoplasm may appear as a rapidly growing tumour, 80% occurring under age four. Known also as a Wilm's tumour it accounts for approximately 8% of childhood malignancies. This tumour spreads rapidly by the blood stream producing metastases in the lungs. Microscopically it is composed of a mass of spindle-shaped cells in which acini and tubules are found.

2. False
Osteogenic sarcoma (osteosarcoma) arises from the cells of the primitive bone-forming mesenchyme. It is the commonest primary malignant tumour of bone excluding myeloma. Seventy-five per cent of sufferers are between 10 and 25 years of age but a similar tumour also occurs in older patients suffering from Paget's disease of bone.

3. True
These tumours develop in the cerebellum forming a soft greyish-white mass which commonly protrudes into the fourth ventricle and spreads over the surface of the brain in a thin sheet to obscure the normal convoluted surface. Microscopically they are composed of spherical or cylindrical cells which have little cytoplasm and no fibrils. Rosettes occur without a central cavity. These tumours are highly malignant but extremely radiosensitive.

4. False
These rare tumours develop from the cells of the biliary epithelium and are less common than true hepatocellular carcinoma. They are commonest in the Far East, in which the majority are associated with infestation by liver flukes.

5. False
An anaplastic squamous carcinoma heavily infiltrated with lymphocytes. This tumour is particularly common in adult Chinese in whom it is commonly associated with a high titre of antibody to the Epstein–Barr virus.

14.14 The following tumours may produce hormones:
1. choriocarcinoma
2. bronchial carcinoma

3. fibroma of the ovary
4. islet cell tumours of the pancreas
5. chromophobe pituitary adenoma

1. True
Choriocarcinoma may be defined as a malignant tumour of trophoblastic origin. Most of these tumours are derived from gestational trophoblast and are a late complication of pregnancy. Non-gestational choriocarcinoma occasionally occurs, usually in the testes or in ovarian teratoma. Associated with pregnancy, approximately 50% arise in hydatidiform moles, 25% following abortions and 20% in a normal pregnancy. The tumours secrete chorionic gonadotrophin and in response to this stimulus ovarian cysts with luteinised theca interna are found in about one third of patients. The secretion of this hormone is an important feature, since failure of the level to fall to normal following treatment with chemotherapy, indicates tumour is still present.

2. True
Bronchogenic carcinoma may secrete a variety of hormones producing thereby a number of 'paraneoplastic syndromes'. The tumour like factors which may be secreted include:
(1) An antidiuretic hormone inducing hyponatraemia
(2) Adrenocorticotrophic hormone causing Cushing's syndrome; this is the commonest hormonal manifestation
(3) Parathyroid related hormone causing hypercalcaemia
(4) Calcitonin causing hypocalcaemia
(5) Gonadotrophins causing gynaecomastia in the male
(6) Serotonin causing the carcinoid syndrome.

3. False
Benign fibromas of the ovary do not produce any hormonal disturbance but large tumours of this type may be associated with wasting, ascites and right sided hydrothorax, Meig's syndrome.

4. True
Islet cell tumours may be entirely non-functional, but if functional they may be associated with either hypoglycaemia due to the excessive and abnormal production of insulin or the Zollinger–Ellison syndrome due to the production of gastrin. This latter is associated with recalcitrant peptic ulceration.

5. True
Chromophobe adenomas constitute about one quarter of all pituitary tumours. Since they are most commonly non-functioning, they produce their effects chiefly by local pressure on adjacent structure, e.g. causing abnormal visual fields. Later, progressive panhypopituitarism develops causing hypothyroidism and hypogonadism. Although lacking clinical effects, immunochemical reactions reveal in some tumours demonstrable FSH and less frequently LH.

SECTION 15. VIRAL DISEASES

15.1 The following are viral diseases:
1. cytomegalic inclusion disease
2. trachoma
3. dengue
4. primary atypical pneumonia
5. typhus

1. True
CMD is caused by a B group herpes virus which, infecting a normal individual, is asymptomatic or causes a mononucleosis-like infection. However, infection by this virus in the neonate or immunosuppressed individual causes serious consequences. In neonates, infection with CMV may cause a condition resembling erythroblastosis foetalis in which severe haemolytic anaemia occurs associated with purpura, hepatosplenomegaly, pneumonitis, deafness and extensive brain damage. In immunosuppressed individuals, the virus causes oesophagitis, colitis, pneumonitis, renal damage, chorioretinitis and meningoencephalitis. In patients already suffering from AIDS, CMV pneumonitis is nearly always associated with infection with *Pneumocytis carinii.*
Cells infected with CMV are markedly enlarged containing large purple staining intranuclear inclusions surrounded by a clear halo.

2. False
Trachoma is a chronic suppurative disease of the eye in which a follicular keratoconjunctivitis develops. It is caused by various subtypes of *Chlamydia trachomatis* and is one of the commonest causes of blindness in the world. It is transmitted by direct human contact or possibly by flies and is commonest in sandy regions and in nomads.

3. True
Dengue is an acute painful febrile illness which is often haemorrhagic. It is produced by an RNA virus of the togavirus type. The virus is arthropod borne (Arbor) and transmitted by the mosquito *Aedes aegypti.* The dengue virus is related to that causing yellow fever.

4. False
Primary atypical pneumonia is caused by the *Mycoplasma pneumoniae* which are 200 to 250 nm in diameter and among the smallest of bacteria. Patients with mycoplasmal pneumonia have autoantibodies against the I antigen carried on erythrocytes.

5. False
Epidemic typhus which is transmitted by the louse, is caused by the *Rickettsia prowazeki*, obligate intracellular parasites that can be grown in tissue culture or eggs. The rickettsiae are small organisms 300 to 700 nm in diameter. Other rickettsiae cause similar febrile illnesses and are either flea or tick borne. The chief microscopic

changes in typhus are seen in the small blood vessels in which proliferation and swelling of the endothelium may cause narrowing. Surrounding the affected vessels is an inflammatory reaction chiefly composed of leucocytes. Thrombosis of affected vessels leads to gangrene of the skin and other areas.

15.2 Encephalitis may be a complication of the following virus infections:
1. Epstein–Barr virus
2. measles virus
3. rubella virus
4. herpes virus
5. adenovirus

1. True
The Epstein–Barr virus is a gamma-group herpes virus normally causing fever, generalized lymph node enlargement, splenomegaly and the appearance in the blood of mononucleosis cells which are atypical activated T lymphocytes. In immune deficient states, infection with this virus causes lymphoma and Burkitt's lymphoma. In normal individuals meningoencephalitis may occur.

2. True
Measles is caused by an RNA virus of the paramyxovirus family and is only rarely a cause of transient encephalitis because most children develop a T cell-mediated immunity controlling the infection. In immunocompromised individuals however, a condition known as subacute sclerosing panencephalitis may occur caused possibly by a hypermutated 'defective' virus that cannot produce either matrix or envelope proteins. The measles virus is spread by droplets and multiplies in the epithelial cells of the upper respiratory tract.

3. True
A progressive encephalitis may occur in children with the congenital rubella syndrome. However its real importance is that it is teratogenic and may cause serious fetal damage. A female infected in the first sixteen weeks of pregnancy has a 1:4 chance of giving birth to a child with some congenital abnormality.

4. True
Herpes simplex infection may be associated with meningo-encephalitis, particularly in immunodepressed individuals.

5. False
The adenoviruses chiefly affect the upper respiratory tract and occasionally cause gastroenteritis. They are not particularly associated with the development of encephalitis.

15.3 Inclusion bodies are found in the following viral infections:
1. measles
2. yellow fever

3. rabies
4. hepatitis B
5. smallpox

1. True
In the hyperplastic lymphoid organs with follicular hyperplasia and large germinal centres, multinucleate giant cells can be found randomly arranged which contain eosinophilic cytoplasmic inclusion bodies. These cells, known as the Warthin–Finkeledy cells, can be found in the sputum and are pathognomonic of the disease.

2. True
Yellow fever is caused by an arbovirus of the B group. The infection is transmitted by the mosquitoe, *Aedes aegypti*. Death is caused by acute hepatic necrosis. Within 72 hours of infection, examination of the liver shows an eosinophilic degeneration of the cytoplasm producing the Councilman bodies. Very occasionally spherical eosinphilic inclusion bodies develop in the nuclei of the affected liver cells called Torres bodies.

3. True
Rabies is caused by rhabdoviruses. The pathognomonic histological feature of this disease is the development of acidophilic cytoplasmic inclusion bodies known as Negri bodies in the neurons, particularly in the pyramidal cells of the hippocampus and in the Purkinje cells in the cerebellum.

4. False
Intracellular inclusion bodies are not found in infections due to the hepatitis B virus. However, actual HBV particles may be found in the serum by electron microscopy.

5. True
Both smallpox and vaccinia are associated with the development of spheroidal eosinophilic masses in the cytoplasm of the epidermal cells known as the Guanieri bodies. Within them the elementary particles of the virus which contain DNA are elaborated.

15.4 The following are DNA containing viruses:
1. rhinovirus
2. herpes virus
3. vaccinia
4. yellow fever
5. influenza

1. False
Rhinoviruses are upper respiratory tract viruses causing the common cold. They are a subgroup of the picornaviruses, a group which also includes the enteroviruses. Their habitat is the nose and they are amongst the smallest of all viruses infecting man.

2. True
The herpes viruses cause herpes simplex, varicella/zoster, cytomegalic inclusion disease and infectious mononucleosis. They are DNA viruses with a capsid of cubical symmetry possessing no outer envelope. Among the most interesting members of this group is the Epstein–Barr virus which is the cause of infectious mononucleosis and is also found in children suffering from Burkitt's lymphoma in Central Africa.

3. True
Vaccinia is a large brick shaped DNA containing virus belonging to the group known as the poxviruses. Included in this group is also the virus responsible for smallpox.

4. False
Yellow fever is caused by an RNA containing togavirus, most of which are arthropod borne, hence the collective name for the group, the ARBOR viruses.

5. False
The Influenza virus is an RNA myxovirus. The capsid has a helical symmetry and an outer envelope. This group of viruses undergo frequent antigenic variations making it difficult to prepare effective vaccines. Epidemic influenza is caused by the subgroup Influenza A.

15.5 The Epstein–Barr virus is associated with:
1. glandular fever
2. the Australia antigen
3. Burkitt's lymphoma
4. nasopharyngeal carcinoma
5. the common cold

1. True
The Epstein–Barr virus (EBV) is a herpes virus. The peripheral lymphocytes in patients suffering from this disease can be shown to contain the virus. Furthermore, during the acute phase of the illness antibodies to EBV can be identified in the patient's serum. In addition individuals suffering from infectious mononucleosis also develop heterophile antibodies in the serum which are capable of agglutinating sheep erythrocytes; such antibodies are not absorbed by guinea-pig kidney but can be absorbed with ox erythrocytes, the basis of the Paul-Bunnell test.

2. False
The Australia antigen is not associated with infection by the EBV. It is associated, however, with the hepatitis B virus and is the name originally given to Hepatitis B surface antigen (HBsAg) because this antigen was originally identified in the serum of an Australian aborigine.

3. True
The EBV was first isolated from cultures of lymphoblasts in children suffering from Burkitt's lymphoma, a tumour affecting the jaws and facial region of children in Central Africa. It is especially prevalent in malaria endemic areas possibly because chronic malarial infection reduces immunity to the virus. An unexplained finding is the relatively low titre of anti-EBV antibodies found in Burkitt's lymphoma.

4. True
Nasopharyngeal carcinoma is associated with a high titre of antibodies to EBV.

5. False
The common cold is associated with rhinoviruses, a subgroup of the picornaviruses.

15.6 The hepatitis B virus:
1. is transmitted by the oral route
2. is transmitted by dogs
3. is common in renal dialysis units
4. is the cause of Burkitt's lymphoma
5. causes immune complex disease

1. True
Hepatitis B virus (HBV) is a DNA virus transmitted by the oral-faecal route, by aerosols or by syringe and needle. An HBV infection can be detected by identifying the antigen HBsAg in the serum of carriers.

2. False
There does not appear to be an intermediate host. However, in the tropics a mosquito vector has been suspected.

3. True
Renal dialysis units are high risk areas for HBV infection as infection is common in people with chronic renal failure. A number of renal units have been associated with a high mortality among doctors and nursing staff from HBV infection. Other groups in which HBV is common are workers in mental hospitals, drug addicts and homosexuals.

4. False
Burkitt's lymphoma is associated with EB virus infection. HBV infection has, however, been associated with primary hepatoma particularly in the tropics.

5. True
HBV infection may be associated with polyarteritis nodosa and arthritis. Immunoglobulin and complement have both been demonstrated in the walls of blood vessels and immune complexes containing HBV have been demonstrated as aggregates in the serum of infected individuals by electron microscopy.

15.7 The following infections may be successfully prevented by the administration of a vaccine:
1. herpes simplex
2. rabies
3. Lassa fever
4. poliomyelitis
5. yellow fever

1. False
No effective vaccine exists against infection by the herpes viruses. Herpes simplex is an infection in which the virus may remain latent for much of the time, probably in nerve cells.

2. True
An effective vaccine against rabies was first produced by Pasteur in the form of an attenuated virus. The risk associated with this and other similar nervous tissue vaccines is of inducing an autoimmune allergic encephalomyelitis. Modern anti-rabies vaccine is prepared from duck embryos and does not carry such a high rate of neurological complications. Recently a vaccine grown in human diploid fibroblasts has been introduced which appears to cause even fewer neurological complications. However local reactions are common, most patients experiencing pain, erythema and induration at the site of the injection. Fever, malaise and myalgia occur in about one third of patients usually after 5–6 doses.

3. False
There is no effective vaccine against Lassa fever which is caused by a virus of the arenavirus group which is prevalent in West Africa.

4. True
The original Salk vaccine consisted of a sterile aqueous suspension of Types 1, 2 and 3 poliovirus grown in cultures of monkey kidney tissue and then inactivated. It is assayed by its ability to promote the production of neutralizing antibodies to each of the three types of virus. Preferred at this time is the use of live attenuated virus, the Sabin vaccine which should not however be administered to immunocompromised individuals or patients receiving corticosteroids.

5. True
Yellow fever vaccine consists of an aqueous suspension of chick embryo tissue infected with a strain of virus known as 17D which is virulent for mice and although avirulent in man retains its immunizing properties. Active immunity is established within 10 days of administration and persists for many years but innoculation is desirable every 10 years or less if travelling in an endemic area.

15.8 The following viral infections are controlled by cell-mediated immunity:
1. herpes simplex
2. cytomegalic inclusion disease

3. poliomyelitis
4. ECHO virus
5. vaccinia

1. True
The herpes simplex virus can cause severe generalized visceral disease in children born with a primary T-lymphocyte deficiency.

2. True
This ubiquitous virus causes a disseminated infection which particularly affects the upper respiratory tract of babies with T-lymphocyte deficiency, adults receiving immunosuppressive drugs and individuals in whom cell-mediated immunity has diminished due to the development of Hodgkin's disease.

3. False
The polioviruses are classified as picornaviruses among which are the echoviruses and the rhinoviruses which cause upper respiratory tract infections. The polio virus causes a non-specific gastroenteritis and in approximately 1:100 of those infected secondarily invades the lower motor neurons to produce a flaccid paralysis. Natural protection from invasion is provided by the MALT system, mucous associated lymphoid tissue, of the gastrointestinal tract which by secreting a humoral immune response of the IgA isotype prevents invasion.

4. False
The ECHO viruses are a subgroup of the picornaviruses, the name standing for 'enteric cytopathogenic human orphan'. This group is responsible for a variety of febrile illnesses including meningitis, respiratory infections, conjunctivitis and diarrhoea. As with the polioviruses it is believed that natural protection is dependent upon the production of an IgA antibody by the gastrointestinal tract.

5. True
The 'reaction of immunity' to vaccinia virus is a delayed hypersensitivity reaction seen when the individual is vaccinated on the second or subsequent occasions. This reaction is T-lymphocyte mediated as is resistance to clinical infection. The presence of immunity is marked by the failure of the individual to develop a 'pock' at the vaccination site.

15.9 Interferons:
1. are cytokines
2. can be produced in response to mitogens
3. are components of the complement system
4. are important in viral infections
5. are a dialysable fraction

1. True
The interferons are a group of proteins whose chief function is to regulate the immune system. Three groups have so far been recognised: IFNα which is made up of a number of variants which

are produced by leucocytes, IFNβ made by fibroblasts and IFN made by T cells.

2. False
Mitogens such as phytohaemoglutinin and concanavalin A stimulate human and mouse T cells resulting in the increased expression of existing surface markers such as the adhesion molecules which allow increased interaction with other cells.

3. False
The complement system is an entirely different group of proteins whose chief function is to protect an individual from bacterial infections by promoting lysis, opsonisation and chemotaxis.

4. True
The interferons provide protection against viral infections by a number of different mechanisms; by the activation of killer cells with the ability to destroy virus infected targets and by direct inhibition of viral replication. The importance of the interferons has been demonstrated in vivo by treating mice with antibodies to murine interferons. Such mice are killed by a dose of virus several hundred times less than the untreated controls.

5. False
The interferons do not pass through a dialysis membrane.

15.10 The following diseases are caused by chlamydia:
   1. yellow fever
   2. lymphogranuloma venereum
   3. mumps
   4. psittacosis
   5. herpes simplex

1. False
Yellow fever is caused by an arthropod borne RNA virus of the togavirus group. It is transmitted by the mosquito, *Aedes aegypti.*

2. True
Lymphogranuloma venereum is caused by a subgroup A chlamydia which is closely related to the chlamydia causing trachoma. The Frei test for LGV is a delayed hypersensitivity skin test.

3. False
Mumps is caused by a paramyxovirus. Typically a bilateral parotitis occurs but in addition there is a high incidence of involvement of central nervous system and occasionally orchitis. Paramyxoviruses are large filamentous double stranded RNA viruses (150 to 220 nm in size).

4. True
Psittacosis is a febrile disease chiefly involving the respiratory tract, caused by a subgroup B chlamydia. It is acquired by inhaling infected aerosols or dust from birds, usually of domestic origin.

5. False

Herpes viruses are double stranded DNA viruses which produce acidophilic intranuclear inclusion bodies. The herpes viruses have the peculiar property of remaining latent for many months or years and then being reactivated by a variety of stimuli, including UV light and febrile illnesses. The herpes group also includes varicella/zoster, the Epstein–Barr virus and cytomegalovirus.

SECTION 16. VASCULAR CONDITIONS

16.1 The chief pathological changes of atherosclerosis are:
1. deposition of lipid in the smooth muscle cells of the intima
2. fragmentation of the internal elastic lamina
3. calcification
4. contraction of the vessel
5. collagen deposition

1. True

It Is the initial deposition of lipid in the smooth muscle cells, macrophages and 'foam' cells which produces the earliest detectable macroscopic changes in the arteries of the intima known as the 'fatty streak'.

2. True

Fragmentation of the internal elastic lamina causes gradually increasing weakness of the arterial wall which is followed by dilatation and aneurysm formation.

3. True

Calcification occurs in the fibrous plaques which develop within the intimal layer. These plaques contain large quantities of cholesterol ester resembling that of the plasma lipoprotein. Calcification is not so pronounced, however, as in the condition known as Monckeberg's sclerosis.

4. False

Decrease in the lumen of an atherosclerotic artery does not occur, because of contraction of the vessel, but follows encroachment by the increasing size of the fibrous plaques or intimal rupture followed by thrombosis.

5. True

During the stage at which fibrous plaques are forming in the wall of the artery large amounts of collagen are deposited in the wall of the artery. In the wall of a normal artery the ratio of collagen to protein is 1:4 whereas in the calcified plaques this ratio may be reduced by an increase in the absolute amount of collagen to less than 1:2.

16.2 Cholesterol is believed to be of great importance in the development of atherosclerosis because:

1. low plasma cholesterol concentrations are associated with relative freedom from atherosclerotic heart disease
2. high concentrations of cholesterol occur in the atherosclerotic plaques
3. patients suffering from steatorrhoea develop atherosclerosis at a younger age than normal individuals
4. diabetes is associated with an increased incidence of atherosclerosis
5. atherosclerosis can be induced in non-human primates by dietary measures which increase the concentration of cholesterol in the plasma

1. True
This has been well established in numerous epidemiological studies.

2. True
Between one third and one half of the calcium-free dry weight of an atherosclerotic plaque is composed of lipid of which more than 70% is cholesterol.

3. False
Patients suffering from steatorrhoea have either normal or subnormal plasma concentrations of cholesterol and theoretically the development of atherosclerosis should be delayed.

4. False
Although diabetes is associated with an increased incidence of atherosclerosis, it can occur even in diabetics with normal levels of lipid. High Density Lipoprotein (HDL) levels are reduced in Type II diabetes, i.e. diabetes of late onset in which no islet cell antibodies are present and the chief feature is insulin resistance, and the risk of atherosclerosis has been shown to be inversely related to their level, in that the higher the level the lower the risk of the disease. Contributory factors in diabetes are believed to be the increased platelet adhesiveness, obesity and hypertension.

5. True
Atherosclerosis can be induced by high cholesterol containing diets in both rabbits and non-human primates.

16.3 The following conditions are associated with hyperlipidaemia:

1. familial hypercholesterolaemia
2. the nephrotic syndrome
3. Von Gierke's syndrome
4. hyperaldosteronism
5. thyrotoxicosis

1. True
Familial hypercholesterolaemia is one of the most frequently encountered Mendelian disorders. Heterozygous individuals with one

mutant gene representing about 1:500 of the population have a 2–3 fold elevation of plasma cholesterol, whilst homozygous individuals may have a 5–6 fold elevation and suffer myocardial infarction due to the complications of atherosclerosis at a comparatively early age.

2. True
Nephrosis is associated with an increase in cholesterol, triglycerides, VLDL, LDL and a decrease in HDL, the latter possibly due to loss in the urine when severe proteinuria is present. The causes of the lipoprotein abnormalities is their increased synthesis in the liver and a decrease in their catabolism.

3. True
Von Gierke's syndrome is the eponymous name for Type I glycogen storage disease, due to an inborn error of metabolism in which a deficiency of the enzyme glucose-6-phosphatase is present. It is associated with a multiplicity of measurable biochemical abnormalities including a high plasma uric acid, cholesterol, total lipids and a low alkaline phosphatase. The clinical picture is dominated by hepatic enlargement and a failure to thrive and an associated hypoglycaemia.

4. False
This hormonal disturbance has no effect on the plasma lipoprotein concentration.

5. False
Thyrotoxicosis is not associated with lipoprotein disturbance unlike hypothyroidism.

16.4 Gangrene is necrosis together with:
1. desiccation
2. colliquative necrosis
3. involvement of a limb
4. infection of the tissue with Gram-positive organisms
5. putrefaction

1. False
Although the clinician refers to dry gangrene when infarction followed by desiccation has occurred, the pathologist does not recognise this as gangrene. The change in colour in 'dry gangrene' is due to alterations in the haemoglobin of the red cells trapped in the infarcted tissues.

2. False
Colliquative necrosis may well occur in gangrene but this is not essential to the pathological definition.

3. False
Gangrene occurs in many places other than a limb, e.g. around the mouth, in the abdominal wall and in the perineum, but is then usually

associated with infection, e.g. by *Clostridia* or microaerophilic streptococci.

4. False
The bacteria responsible for the specific condition of gas gangrene are Gram-positive.

5. True
Necrosis with superadded putrefaction is the accepted pathological definition of gangrene. The responsible organisms are saprophytic, i.e. grow on decaying organic matter. The organisms concerned include the clostridia (Gram-positive), the bacterioides (Gram-negative) and fusobacterium (Gram-negative).

16.5 Infarction may occur as a complication in the following diseases:
1. atherosclerosis
2. Monckeberg's sclerosis
3. benign hypertension
4. sickle-cell anaemia
5. idiopathic thrombocytopenic purpura

1. True
Infarction may occur in any organ or tissue supplied by an atherosclerotic artery. It is caused by the sudden obstruction to the blood flow by occlusion of the lumen of the artery. This follows a subintimal haemorrhage in the wall of the diseased artery or thrombosis upon the intimal plaque. Typical infarcts of this nature occur in the heart, brain and limbs.

2. False
This is a condition affecting the major arteries of the lower limb in elderly people caused by dystrophic calcification of the media. The intima is unaffected and the lumen of the artery remains of normal diameter unless coincidental atherosclerotic changes have also occurred in the involved blood vessels.

3. False
Hypertension does not lead to infarction unless accompanied by atherosclerosis. In the brain hypertension may be associated with the development of microaneurysms of the deep penetrating arteries. These tend to rupture causing cerebral haemorrhage.

4. True
Sickle-cell anaemia is frequently complicated by vascular occlusive episodes which lead to infarcts in the lungs, spleen, bone, liver or intestine. In severe cases these episodes occur within the first few years of life but they do not occur in the newborn, however severe the disease, because of the high complement of fetal haemoglobin and low percentage of HbS in the erythrocytes.

5. False
ITP occurs chiefly in children and young adults and is frequently a
self-limiting disease which improves within three months. This
condition is associated with bleeding from the endometrium,
kidneys or gastrointestinal tract if the platelet count is below
200 000 per µml.

**16.6 Liquefaction associated with necrosis occurs after infarction of
the:**
1. heart
2. kidney
3. brain
4. liver
5. spleen

1. False
2. False
3. True
4. False
5. False

In the heart, kidney, liver and spleen coagulative necrosis occurs.
The necrotic area becomes swollen, firm, dull and lustreless.
Histologically the outlines of the dead cells are usually visible under a
light microscope and the dead tissue becomes firm because of the
action of tissue thromboplastins on fibrinogen which, together with
other plasma proteins, diffuse from the damaged membranes of the
necrotic cells.

In contrast brain tissue, which has a large fluid component,
becomes 'softened' when necrotic and finally turns into a turbid
liquid. The histological architecture of the affected tissue is lost. This
is colliquative necrosis.

**16.7 The investigations performed in a patient suffering from
Raynaud's phenomenon should include:**
1. assay of haemagglutinating antibodies
2. rheumatoid factor
3. antimitochondrial antibodies
4. serum potassium
5. X-ray of the root of the neck

1. True
This investigation may reveal the presence of cold agglutinins which
by agglutinating the red cells in the digital circulation cause
Raynaud's phenomenon.

2. True
Rheumatoid arthritis may be associated with or mimic Raynaud's
phenomenon. The serum in the majority of patients suffering from

rheumatoid disease contains an IgM immunoglobulin which is an autoantibody reacting with the patient's own IgG. This factor is normally detected by the use of the Waaler–Rose test.

3. False
Antimitochondrial antibodies are found in a number of autoimmune conditions including Hashimoto's disease of the thyroid, known also as lymphadenoid goitre or autoimmune thyroiditis. They are not found associated with Raynaud's phenomenon.

4. False
The serum potassium remains normal in all conditions associated with the Raynaud's phenomenon.

5. True
Raynaud's phenomenon may be associated with a cervical rib. If present, such a rib injures the subclavian artery and causes intimal thrombosis. Embolisation from this thrombus may then cause the vascular changes associated with Raynaud's phenomenon.

16.8 Acquired syphilis of the cardiovascular system may involve the following lesions:
1. myocardial gummata
2. aortitis
3. aortic regurgitation
4. abdominal aortic aneurysm
5. stenosis of the coronary ostia

1. True
Gummata are ubiquitous, occurring in any tissue of the body. A second type of myocardial lesion has been described in which only fibrosis occurs. There is, however, doubt as to whether this represents a specific form of syphilitic involvement.

2. True
The distinctive features of syphilitic aortitis, which is often accompanied by atherosclerosis, are as follows:
    (a) Bluish grey or porcelain-grey intimal plaques
    (b) Wrinkling and puckering of the inner aspect of the aorta with a tendency to form radial or parallel grooves, the latter in the long axis of the aorta
    (c) Sharp transverse demarcation of the aortic lesions ending at the origins of the vessels of the neck, at the level of the diaphragm or at the origin of the renal arteries
    (d) Localization of the most extensive lesions to the ascending aorta above the sinuses of Valsalva.

3. True
Syphilis produces endarteritis of the vasa vasorum with resulting ischaemia of the aortic wall. This causes destruction of the medial elastic leading to weakening of the wall of the aorta and loss of its

elasticity. Since the disease chiefly affects the root of the aorta, the aortic ring widens separating the aortic cusps thus causing aortic regurgitation.

4. False
Abdominal aortic aneurysms are most commonly due to atherosclerosis. Syphilitic aneurysms chiefly occur in the root and ascending parts of the aorta.

5. True
The ostia of the coronary arteries are usually involved in either inflammatory or fibrotic changes which results in narrowing leading to angina pectoris.

16.9 Coarctation of the aorta is associated with:
1. a primary developmental anomaly of the third left aortic arch
2. the development of a collateral circulation to overcome the effects of the abnormality
3. a bicuspid aortic valve
4. hypertension
5. erosion of the upper borders of the ribs

1. False
The embryological abnormality involves the fourth left aortic arch.

2. True
Massive collaterals develop, sometimes limited to within the chest, but in other cases obvious in the subcutaneous tissues.

3. True
In 50% of cases a bicuspid aortic valve is present.

4. False
The hypertension is limited to the upper extremities; the blood pressure in the lower limbs is either normal or below normal.

5. False
The erosions involve the lower borders of the ribs, usually from the third to the tenth; commonly they are bilateral and in the posterior section. They are caused by enlargement of the intercostal vessels.

16.10 The following congenital anomalies of the heart are accompanied by continuous cyanosis:
1. complete transposition of the great vessels
2. uncomplicated patent ductus arteriosus
3. coarctation of the aorta
4. double aortic arch
5. tetralogy of Fallot

1. True

This is one of the leading causes of death from cyanotic heart disease of congenital origin. The aorta arises entirely from the right ventricle and the pulmonary artery from the left.

2. False

In children suffering from uncomplicated patent ductus arteriosus blood at the high pressure in the aorta is shunted into the pulmonary artery during both systole and diastole. The pulmonary blood flow is above normal and the pulmonary artery becomes dilated, cyanosis does not develop until heart failure occurs although occasionally a reversal of flow with venous-arterial shunting may occur during crying or coughing.

3. False

Cyanosis does not occur in this condition. A striking collateral circulation develops but if this is inadequate congestive heart failure develops due to the severe obstruction to blood flow.

4. False

Symptoms from a double aortic arch are often absent. If they occur they consist of dysphagia and dyspnoea.

5. True

This combination of cardiac abnormalities consists of a ventricular septal defect, obstruction to the right ventricular outflow, an aorta which over-rides the VSD and lastly right ventricular hypertrophy. The clinical consequences depend primarily on the severity of the subpulmonary stenosis. It is nearly always associated with cyanosis from birth and accounts for the majority of infants suffering from cyanotic heart disease.

16.11 Acute heart failure occurs:

1. in rheumatic fever
2. in rheumatoid arthritis
3. in myxoedema
4. following myocardial infarction
5. in acute nephritis

1. True

In acute rheumatic fever the pericardium, myocardium and the valves may be affected. In the presence of pericarditis or valvular disease one can virtually assume that myocardial involvement has occurred and evidence of right and left heart failure are commonly observed in children. Cardiac enlargement may occur rapidly in active rheumatic disease. The characteristic lesion is the Aschoff body which when fully developed shows hyaline change in the collagen bundles surrounded by an infiltrate of lymphocytes, macrophages and occasional polymorphonuclear cells. These occur more commonly on the left side of the heart and are especially abundant beneath the endocardium of the left atrium just above the mitral cusp. In addition to this specific lesion diffuse polymorphonuclear and lymphocytic infiltration occurs along the connective tissue planes associated with inflammatory oedema.

2. False
Rheumatoid arthritis has no effect on the heart.

3. False
Although the heart shadow is seen to be enlarged in myxoedema on plain radiographs this is chiefly due to the development of a pericardial effusion. Heart failure does not occur unless there is associated intrinsic heart disease.

4. True
Acute heart failure occurs following severe myocardial infarction due to the reduction in cardiac output resulting from the myocardial injury or the development of ventricular fibrillation.

5. True
Acute nephritis may be followed by heart failure due to the development of severe hypertension associated with this disease. This causes left ventricular failure.

16.12 Left-sided heart failure occurs as a complication of:
1. hypertension
2. mitral regurgitation
3. pulmonary fibrosis
4. uncomplicated coronary atherosclerosis
5. tricuspid stenosis

1. True
Hypertension, depending upon its severity and the rapidity of its onset, places an increasing strain on the myocardium and inevitably left-sided heart failure develops.

2. True
Mitral regurgitation, when it is severe enough to become symptomatic, is associated with palpitations and dyspnoea. In severe cases dyspnoea on slight exertion occurs accompanied by increasing fatigue. In some patients no important manifestations of the condition occur but even so in some of these patients rapidly progressive cardiac failure may develop particularly if a bacterial endocarditis occurs.

3. False
Pulmonary fibrosis places a strain on the right side of the heart.

4. True
Uncomplicated coronary atherosclerosis is asymptomatic. Symptoms will only develop when the disease is sufficiently severe to lead to myocardial fibrosis.

5. False

Tricuspid stenosis is associated with right-sided heart failure.

16.13 A myocardial infarct may be associated with:

1. hypotension
2. a fall in the plasma GOT
3. endocardial thrombosis
4. a red infarct
5. atrial rather than ventricular fibrillation

1. True

A severe myocardial infarct causes a dramatic fall in cardiac output and so 'cardiogenic shock'.

2. False

Since the enzyme glutamic oxaloacetic transaminase is present in heart muscle myocardial necrosis leads to the liberation of this enzyme and an increase in its concentration in the blood. GOT estimations are, therefore, diagnostically useful. Elevated levels which reach a peak within 2 to 3 days can be found within 6 to 12 hours of infarction.

3. True

When the infarct involves the endocardium some thrombosis is almost inevitable. This leads to the possibility of an embolic complication although this is not very common.

4. False

Because the myocardium has only a single arterial supply via the coronary vessels, a pale infarct occurs. No visible changes occur in the dead muscle for 8 hours or more. Therefore, in patients dying within a few hours neither with the naked eye nor under the light microscope can changes be seen.

5. False

The arrhythmia commonly associated with myocardial infarction is ventricular fibrillation. Because the fibrillating ventricle cannot expel blood from its cavity in sufficient volume to sustain life sudden death may follow even a minor infarct.

SECTION 17. HAEMATOLOGY

17.1 A low mean corpuscular haemoglobin concentration occurs in the following:

1. iron deficiency anaemia
2. pernicious anaemia
3. the anaemia associated with infestation with the fish tapeworm
   Diphyllobothrium latum

4. the anaemia following extensive gastric resection
5. sideroblastic anaemia

1. True
Iron deficiency arising from a decreased intake of iron or chronic blood loss leads to a reduction in the MCHC. The common causes of chronic blood loss in the Western World include severe haemorrhoids or menorrhagia. In tropical countries ankylostomiasis is one of the commonest causes of alimentary blood loss.

2. False
The MCHC is normal. The macrocytic red cells vary in shape and size and are well filled with haemoglobin in the absence of a co-existent iron deficiency.

3. False
Diphyllobothrium latum, the fish tapeworm, is common in Scandinavian countries. Infestation causes a pure vitamin B_{12} deficiency by the deviation of the vitamin from the host to the parasite.

4. True
Extensive gastric resection may be followed by an anaemia in which the MCHC falls because both vitamin B_{12} and iron absorption may be disturbed.

5. False
Sideroblastic anaemia results from the defective synthesis of haem. The chief laboratory finding is found in the marrow erythroblasts in which a perinuclear ring of iron granules develops. The condition may occur as a rare congenital disorder when it is transmitted as a sex linked recessive disorder and is thus uncommon in women, or it may be acquired. In acquired disease, no cause can be found in 50% of patients and in the others a variety of drugs have been implicated including PAS, paracetamol and phenacetin. Most cases are however due to malnutrition, commonly caused by chronic alcoholism or a previous gastric operation. The MCHC is not markedly depressed and the plasma iron is either normal or raised, thus differentiating the condition from an iron deficiency anaemia.

17.2 Alterations in the structure of the Hb molecule give rise to the following diseases:
1. haemolytic disease of the newborn
2. sickle-cell anaemia
3. paroxysmal cold haemoglobinuria
4. paroxysmal nocturnal haemoglobinuria
5. thalassaemia major

1. False
This condition is due to the stimulation of maternal antibody production by an antigen possessed by the fetus and is unrelated to

the actual structure of the haemoglobin molecule. The common situation is of a mother Rh-d carrying a fetus Rh-D. Isoimmunization initially occurs in the immediate post-partum phase of placental separation in the first pregnancy. The mother is then sensitized. Any subsequent pregnancy in which the fetus is Rh positive leads to recurrent antibody production. Haemolysis of the fetal red cells is then brought about by the transplacental passage of maternal antibody into the fetal circulation.

2. True
Sickle-cell anaemia is a hereditary condition of Negroes transmitted by an autosome. The homozygous condition gives rise to the severe sickle-cell disease, the heterozygous condition the sickle-cell trait. The abnormal haemoglobin is known as Hb-S which reduced in a low oxygen tension becomes insoluble. This causes the red cells to assume a bizarre shape and become prone to haemolysis. In addition the sickled red cells block the capillaries to produce infarcts, particularly in the spleen and bones.

3. False
This disorder may be associated either with a haemolysin or haemagglutinin, the antibody having maximum activity below body temperature, usually at about 20°C. Thus acute intravascular lysis occurs after exposure of the whole or part of the body to cold.

4. False
Although known as PNH, in only about 25% of patients does the condition present in the classical manner i.e. with paroxysmal attacks of haemolysis occurring at night. In the majority the condition presents as a chronic iron deficiency anaemia, due to chronic haemolysis accompanied by loss of iron in the urine. It may also be associated with venous thromboses involving the hepatic, portal or cerebral veins. The condition is due to a somatic mutation of a pluripotential stem cell causing the progeny of these cells, i.e. red cells, white cells and platelets to be deficient in a family of proteins attached to the cell membrane by gylcosylphosphatidylinositol anchors. These GPI linked proteins inactivate complement and their absence renders the red cells unusually sensitive to lysis by endogenous complement.

5. True
Thalassaemia major is the homozygous form of this disorder in which synthesis of the α or β chains of the haemoglobin molecule is defective. The condition often presents as an apparent haemolytic anaemia of infancy accompanied by pallor and splenomegaly, and the mean red cell survival time is grossly reduced.

17.3 The following are haemoglobinopathies:
  1. congenital spherocytosis
  2. sickle-cell anaemia
  3. thalassaemia

4. cold Agglutination Immune Haemolytic Anaemia
5. eliptocytosis

1. False
Congenital spherocytosis is a condition in which a defect in the red cell membrane is present, chiefly due to a deficiency of spectrin, the major protein of the membrane. This causes a reduction in the stability of the cell membrane with the result that the red cells assume a spherical shape which thus reduces membrane plasticity. Such cells have great difficulty in passing through the cords of Billroth in the spleen which requires considerable deformity of the red cells to accomplish. Thus the affected cells are trapped in the spleen and by being unable to extrude sodium, are subjected to osmotic damage at which point they are totally destroyed by mononuclear cells.

2. True
Sickle-cell anaemia is due to a point mutation that leads to substitution of valine for glutamic acid at the sixth position of the β globin chain. The result is the formation of HbS which, on deoxygenation, undergoes aggregation and polymerization leading to physical change in the haemoglobin which causes the red cell to be distorted, becoming sickle shaped. Initially the condition is reversible, but after repeated attacks they remain distorted and are then haemolysed.

3. True
There are numerous thalassaemia syndromes but all are basically due to a decreased synthesis of either the α or β globin chain of HbA (α2 β2). When all four chains are deleted, the condition of hydrops fotalis develops in which the excess of gamma-globulin chains form tetramers (Hb Barts) which, although having a high affinity for oxygen, are unable to deliver it to the tissues. Severe tissue anoxia results in intrauterine fetal death. In β thalassaemia major, children suffer growth defects and die at an early age due to anaemia. Other than these two extreme conditions, there are a huge number of variants depending on the type of genetic defect. Thus a silent carrier state can occur in which there is little reduction in α chain synthesis; such individuals carry 3 normal α globin genes.

4. False
This condition may occur in:
    (1) an acute form during the recovery phase from an acute infection.
    (2) a chronic form in lymphoproliferative disorders.
    (3) an idiopathic condition.

It is caused by the development of IgM antibodies which bind to red cells at low temperatures between 0–4°C, hence the term 'cold agglutinins'. The condition causes a haemolytic anaemia of varying severity; in severe cases immediate haemolysis occurs, whereas in others the IgM bound to the red cells is released at normal temperatures but leaves complement C3b bound to the red cell membranes, making these cells susceptible to phagocytosis by the mononuclear cells in the spleen and liver.

5. False

Eliptocytosis is a hereditary disorder in which a large proportion of the red cells are oval in shape. Like hereditary spherocytosis, it is due to an abnormality of the red cell cytoskeleton leading to trapping and destruction of the affected cells in the cords of Billroth in the spleen.

17.4 Iron deficiency anaemia may be associated with the following:
1. a sensitive and painful glossitis
2. dysphagia
3. a rise in the liver iron
4. koilonychia
5. chlorosis

1. False

A sensitive, painful glossitis is typical of vitamin B_{12} and folate deficiency although chronic iron deficiency leads to atrophy of the tongue papillae.

2. True

Dysphagia is a rare association with chronic iron deficiency. This combination is known as the Plummer–Vinson or Patterson–Kelly syndrome, a characteristic feature of which is the development of dysphagia due either to neuromuscular incoordination of the upper end of the oesophagus or the development of webs at the same level.

3. False

Demonstrable changes in iron metabolism develop before the Hb begins to fall. The first change is a depletion of the body stores of iron. This can be demonstrated either by liver biopsy or from specimens of aspirated bone marrow.

4. True

This is one of the characteristic features of severe iron deficiency anaemia. The nails of the radial fingers of the hand show the most pronounced changes; they become brittle and tend to split. Later they soften, become flatter and later even concave. Koilonychia is most marked in patients who immerse their hands in water.

5. True

This condition which is now no longer seen was first described in the sixteenth century. Chlorosis occurred in adolescent girls suffering from severe iron deficiency anaemia and was marked by the development of a yellowish or greenish complexion. The probable aetiology was a combination of a poor diet, rapid growth and the onset of menstruation.

17.5 The production of red blood cells is depressed by the following conditions:
1. chronic renal failure
2. excessive administration of glucocorticoids
3. subacute rheumatic fever
4. myxoedema
5. disseminated breast cancer

1. True
Chronic renal failure is invariably associated with anaemia. This is believed to be due to marrow depression probably caused by the inadequate production of erythropoietin. The severity of the anaemia, however, does not always coincide with the degree of uraemia.

2. False
The administration of excessive quantities of glucocorticoids has little effect on erythropoiesis except indirectly as changes in the plasma volume occur. However, in Cushing's disease a mild erythrocytosis may be present.

3. True
Anaemia is a common complication of subacute rheumatic fever in childhood particularly when the disease is accompanied by joint pains and active carditis.

4. True
In animals a normocytic, normochromic anaemia follows removal of the thyroid, the anaemia being corrected by the administration of thyroxine. In man the severity of the anaemia in myxoedema and its frequency vary according to the series examined. However, thyroid deficiency should always be considered in the differential diagnosis when a normocytic anaemia fails to respond to treatment.

5. True
Red cell production is depressed in disseminated breast cancer when the red marrow is replaced by malignant tissue.

17.6 Pathological destruction of red blood cells can take place in the following sites:
1. the submucosal plexus of the small intestine
2. the peripheral circulation
3. the liver
4. the spleen
5. the bone marrow

1. False
2. True
3. True
4. True
5. True

Pathological red cell destruction occurs in two major sites, either within the peripheral circulation when the contents of the erythrocyte are liberated into the plasma or secondly, in intimate proximity to the cells of the mononuclear-phagocyte system (3.4.5), a system previously known as the reticuloendothelial system. In the latter sites the products of red cell destruction can be immediately phagocytosed.

Intravascular haemolysis can be caused by a number of factors which include:
(a) Toxic substances such as lead, benzene and phenylhydrazine
(b) Parasitic infections such as malaria
(c) Invasive bacterial infections causing septicaemia
(d) Following burns

Extravascular haemolysis is chiefly seen:
(a) In the presence of structural abnormalities of the red cell, e.g. congenital spherocytosis and thalassaemia
(b) When incomplete agglutinating antibodies are present in the circulation, e.g. in diffuse lupus erythematosus or ulcerative colitis
(c) In the presence of diseases of the mononuclear-phagocyte system (reticuloendothelial system), e.g. Hodgkin's lymphoma

The submucosal plexus of the gastrointestinal tract plays no part in the destruction of red cells.

17.7 The commonest haemolytic disorder in the world is:
1. congenital spherocytosis
2. disseminated lupus erythematosus
3. malaria
4. G6PD deficiency
5. sickle disease

The correct answer is **3**. All the conditions listed cause haemolysis but malaria is the commonest of them all because of its widespread distribution. Haemolysis occurs in malaria due to parasitisation of the red cells by the merozoites which then go through further cycles of asexual proliferation until the red cell is destroyed. This occurs with every bout of fever.

17.8 The following haemolytic disorders are congenital:
1. thalassaemia
2. march haemoglobinuria
3. microangiopathic haemolytic anaemia
4. ovalocytosis
5. G6PD deficiency

1. True
Thalassaemia is a complex disorder in which the main abnormality is a defect in the synthesis of one of the polypeptide chains of the

globin of haemoglobin A. Heterozygotes show some evidence of mild haemolytic disease, thalassaemia minor, whereas homozygotes are severely affected and seldom survive beyond early adult life.

2. False
This condition of acute haemoglobinuria, usually mild, results from long marches. Haemolysis is believed to be caused by mechanical damage to the red cells as they flow through the plantar aspect of the feet during long marches on hard surfaces.

3. False
This condition is the result of disseminated intravascular coagulation and occurs in a variety of conditions including disseminated malignancy, fulminating septicaemia and the haemolytic uraemic syndrome. Severe haemolytic anaemia occurs associated with distortion and fragmentation of the red cells.

4. True
Ovalocytosis is a hereditary condition in which a high proportion of red cells are ovalocytes and many develop a rod-shaped deformity. The condition is transmitted as an autosomal dominant.

5. True
G6PD deficiency is a rare condition in which the life span of the red cells is shortened. G6PD is concerned with the maintenance of the NADP/NADPH ratio so that the majority of glutathione in the red cell is in the reduced state. How this substance maintains the integrity of the red cell membrane is unknown.

17.9 Congenital spherocytosis is a haemolytic disorder:
1. inherited as an autosomal recessive
2. associated with chronic anaemia
3. basically caused by a developmental defect of the red cell membrane
4. associated with massive enlargement of the spleen
5. in which the osmotic fragility of the red cell is diminished

1. False
Hereditary spherocytosis is inherited as an autosomal dominant of variable penetrance, the latter determining the clinical severity of the disease.

2. True
The majority of patients suffering from hereditary spherocytosis suffer from chronic anaemia, although some patients do not develop symptoms until adult life.

3. True
The fundamental defect in congenital spherocytosis is in the red cell membrane which diminishes the plasticity of the red cells and thus their deformability in the cords of Billroth in the spleen. This is due to a deficiency in one or more of the proteins of which the membrane is

composed, but especially in the spectrin content which may be reduced by as much as 50%. It is this defect which causes the cell to assume a spherical shape, in which conformation it is trapped in the spleen. There, unable to prevent the passive influx of Na+ ion due to loss of ATP, they undergo osmotic injury followed by total destruction by the mononuclear cells.

4. False
This condition is associated with only moderate enlargement of the spleen. The spherocytes characteristic of this disease are trapped in the cords of Billroth.

5. False
Osmotic fragility is enhanced in congenital spherocytosis. It is this abnormality which led to the recognition of the disease towards the end of the nineteenth century.

17.10 Polycythaemia occurs in:
1. congenital cyanotic heart disease
2. tumours of the renal parenchyma, renal carcinoma
3. the carcinoid syndrome
4. lead poisoning
5. hypoxia

1. True
Intense polycythaemia is frequently present in congenital heart disease with the result that the blood volume is increased, primarily due to an increase in red cell volume. In consequence the haematocrit is high (see 5).

2. True
Polycythaemia occurs in association with renal carcinoma because of the high output of erythropoietin by some of these tumours.

3. False
The plethoric appearance of the face in the carcinoid syndrome which might suggest polycythaemia is due to telangiectasia of the skin together with release of the enzyme kallikrein from the tumour which produces bradykinin from plasma substrates.

4. False
Lead poisoning produces chronic anaemia which probably depends upon two factors:
    (a) Interference with synthesis of haemoglobin
    (b) Excessive fragility of the red cells

5. True
Hypoxia of any type, especially that associated with chronic respiratory insufficiency, congenital heart disease with right to left shunts, or living at high altitudes is a common cause of secondary polycythaemia. The bone marrow is stimulated by erythropoietin.

17.11 Megaloblastic anaemia may be caused by:
1. atrophy or ablation of the gastric mucosa
2. infestation with *Diphyllobothrium latum*
3. lesions involving the terminal ileum
4. over enthusiastic use of purgatives
5. small bowel blind loops

1. True
Atrophy of the gastric mucosa is the underlying cause of classic pernicious anaemia. Ablation of the gastric mucosa by total gastrectomy will lead to a megaloblastic anaemia after the natural reserves of B_{12} in the liver have been exhausted in about 3 to 4 years.

2. True
This helminth competes with the host for vitamin B_{12}. This type of megaloblastic anaemia is found only in Finland despite the world wide distribution of the worm.

3. True
The lesion may be inflammatory as in Crohn's disease or the bowel may have been resected. A megaloblastic anaemia follows because the terminal ileum is the site of absorption of vitamin B_{12} and folic acid.

4. False
Purgatives act on the colon which is not concerned with the absorption of vitamin B_{12} or folic acid.

5. True
Small bowel blind loops may be the result of a surgical procedure, e.g. jejunal resection followed by side to side or an end to side anastomosis. This causes a megaloblastic anaemia because the intrinsic factor-B_{12} complex normally formed in the stomach fails to reach its absorptive site in the distal ileum. This is due to the abnormal proliferation of bacteria in such loops which compete for and take up the IF-B_{12} complex. A similar situation may develop in patients suffering from jejunal diverticulosis.

17.12 The following abnormalities occur in pernicious anaemia:
1. a low haemoglobin
2. a decreased mean corpuscular haemoglobin (MCH)
3. an increased reticulocyte count
4. antibodies to the parietal cells
5. a decrease in the circulating level of vitamin B_{12}

1. True
The definition of anaemia is a fall in the number of red cells or quantity of haemoglobin in a given volume of blood in the presence of a low or normal total blood volume. In pernicious anaemia the number of red cells is diminished but the plasma volume increases.

2. False
The mean corpuscular haemoglobin is elevated and the mean corpuscular volume is greater than normal although individual cells show great variation in size.

3. False
It may be normal but rises rapidly once treatment begins. In percentage terms the reticulocyte count may rise within a week following a single intramuscular injection of vitamin B_{12} from 3 to 50.

4. True
Three types of antibody may be found in patients suffering from pernicious anaemia. In approximately three quarters, a 'blocking' antibody of IgG type can be found which blocks the binding of vitamin B_{12} to the intrinsic factor; a second antibody known as a 'binding' antibody is found in about half the patients, which reacts with both the intrinsic factor and vitamin B_{12} and thirdly, in about 90% of all sufferers, an antibody can be found localized in the microvilli of the canalicular system of the gastric parietal cells, referred to as the parietal canalicular antibody, which is directed against the proton pump. Despite the presence of these antibodies, it has not been precisely established that they are the cause of the mucosal atrophy.

5. True
Vitamin B_{12}, the extrinsic factor, cannot be absorbed in the absence of the intrinsic factor (IF) which is produced by the parietal cells. Hence in classical pernicious anaemia the serum vitamin B_{12} is reduced.

17.13 In pernicious anaemia the following pathological changes may be seen:
1. haemosiderosis
2. atrophy of the gastric mucosa
3. a decrease in the volume of red marrow in the long bones
4. extramedullary haemopoiesis
5. demyelination of the lateral and dorsal columns, not associated with gliosis

1. True
Haemosiderin is ferritin with an iron content of about 36%. This pigment forms brown insoluble granules which give the Prussian blue reaction. Haemosiderosis occurs in pernicious anaemia because of haemolysis and the diversion of the iron normally present in the circulating haemoglobin to the tissues.

2. True
The mucosa of the stomach shows a generalized atrophic change with almost complete destruction of the specialized cells of the fundus including the parietal cells which are replaced by mucus secreting cells resembling those lining the large intestine.

3. False
Increasing erythropoiesis leads to an extension of the red marrow.

4. True
In severe pernicious anaemia foci of ectopic erythropoiesis can be found in the liver and spleen.

5. True
This change, known as subacute combined degeneration, occurs only in pure vitamin B_{12} deficiency. It does not occur in folic acid deficiency. The principal changes occur in the spinal cord in which degeneration of the myelin of the dorsal and lateral tracts occurs sometimes followed by axonal loss. Clinically these changes result in a spastic paresis, sensory ataxia and severe parasthesia in the lower limbs. Less commonly degenerative changes are seen in the posterior ganglia, this giving rise to the term 'combined degeneration'.

17.14 The following biochemical changes occur in pernicious anaemia:
1. a raised serum vitamin B_{12}
2. a normal serum folate
3. a raised serum bilirubin
4. an increased alkaline phosphatase
5. a decreased plasma copper

1. False
The reverse is true, the serum vitamin B_{12} falls due to decreased absorption. This is caused by an absence of the intrinsic factor which is normally formed by the stomach. In pernicious anaemia a diffuse atrophic gastritis occurs.

2. True
In classical pernicious anaemia the serum folate levels are normal although the histidine test may produce abnormal FIGLU excretion.

3. True
In classical pernicious anaemia haemolysis occurs. This is sufficient to cause a slight elevation of the serum bilirubin, an increase in the amount of stercobilinogen in the faeces and moderate urobilinuria.

4. False
Alkaline phosphatase plays no part in the metabolism of haemoglobin.

5. False
Although copper is essential for normal erythropoiesis no changes occur in the concentration of this in the serum in pernicious anaemia.

17.15 An absolute lymphocytosis occurs in the following conditions:
1. extensive skin diseases such as psoriasis, eczema, pemphigus

2. Löeffler's syndrome
3. tuberculosis
4. pertussis
5. chronic lymphatic leukaemia

1. False
Chronic and extensive skin diseases such as those named in the question are not associated with a lymphocytosis.

2. False
Löeffler's syndrome is a pulmonary eosinophilia which is associated with a hypersensitivity state in which the commonest allergen is a worm such as *Ascaris lumbricoides*. Many other factors have been implicated including several drugs such as para-aminosalicylic acid and chlorpropamide. An eosinophilia occurs but this is not associated with a lymphocytosis. Clinically a cough develops and transient areas of infiltration may be seen in plain radiographs of the chest.

3. True
Chronic infections such as tuberculosis and syphilis may be accompanied by an absolute lymphocytosis.

4. True
Whooping cough is accompanied by a marked lymphocytosis even before the classical whoop has developed, counts as high as 100 000 per μl may be found.

5. True
In chronic lymphatic leukaemia the absolute lymphocyte count may exceed 100 000 per μl. The majority of cells appear to be normal mature small lymphocytes but larger more primitive cells are also found. In many cases the leukaemic lymphocytes possess surface immunoglobulins characteristic of B cells.

17.16 Acute myeloblastic leukaemia:
1. is most common in young adults
2. is associated with the presence of a large number of primitive cells in the marrow and peripheral blood
3. is associated with peripheral white counts in excess of 100 000 per μl
4. may be associated with a normal white count
5. marrow aspirates show decreased cellularity

1. False
The highest incidence of acute myeloid leukaemia occurs between 30–50 years of age similar in fact to the greatest incidence of the chronic form of the disease. This is in contrast to acute lymphocytic forms in which the greatest incidence occurs before the age of 10 years.

2. True
In acute leukaemias the predominant cell in the marrow or blood is the myeloblast, lymphoblast or monoblast according to the type of leukaemia.

3. False
In acute leukaemia the total white count is only moderately raised, counts between 20 000 and 50 000 per µl being common. In contrast in the various forms of chronic leukaemia the peripheral white count may exceed 300 000 per µl.

4. True
In over one-third of all cases the total white count is normal or even reduced, so-called aleukaemic leukaemia. However, even in these cases primitive cells can almost always be found in the peripheral blood.

5. False
The typical picture in acute leukaemia is an increase in cellularity. Sections of the marrow show replacement of the fat spaces by primitive leukaemic cells.

17.17 Myeloid metaplasia is associated with:
1. a variable peripheral white count
2. extramedullary haemopoiesis
3. the Philadelphia chromosome
4. a decreased number of megakaryocytes in the marrow
5. anaemia

1. True
The white cell count in the peripheral blood may range from 3000 to 30 000 per µl.

2. True
The term myeloid metaplasia is used to describe extramedullary haemopoiesis which occurs chiefly in the spleen and liver and only rarely in other organs.

3. False
The Philadelphia chromosome, a deletion of the long arms of one of the chromosome 22 pair in the white cell, is found in 90% of sufferers from chronic myeloid leukaemia. It is not found in myeloid metaplasia.

4. False
One of the characteristic features of myeloid metaplasia is the presence of an increased number of megakaryocytes in the bone marrow.

5. True
Myeloid metaplasia may be associated with either anaemia or polycythaemia, the former is occasionally sufficiently severe to require blood transfusion.

17.18 Chronic myeloid leukaemia is associated with:

1. the presence of large numbers of myeloblasts in the peripheral blood
2. a very variable total white count
3. massive splenomegaly
4. lymph nodes enlargement
5. hepatomegaly

1. False
The dominant white cell in the peripheral circulation is the neutrophil myelocyte and only a few myeloblasts are present.

2. True
The white count may vary between 15 000 and 500 000 per μl. Sufficient mature cells are usually present to make the diagnosis without difficulty.

3. True
Massive splenomegaly occurs because this organ becomes infiltrated by myelocytes and polymorphonuclear leucocytes. Pale infarcts are common.

4. False
In chronic myeloid leukaemia the lymph nodes are usually normal in size in contrast to the situation in chronic lymphatic leukaemia in which the lymph nodes are usually enlarged early in the course of the disease.

5. True
In chronic myeloid leukaemia primitive cells are found in the sinusoids. In contrast in chronic lymphocytic leukaemia the primitive cells infiltrate the periportal areas.

17.19 Chronic myeloid leukaemia differs from chronic lymphatic leukaemia in that:

1. in the former the predominant white cell in the circulation is the leucocyte
2. the total white count is higher in chronic lymphatic leukaemia
3. in the former the proliferating marrow cells possess the Philadelphia chromosome
4. the latter is more common in an older age group than is the former
5. the former disease tends to develop into a more aggressive type of acute leukaemia

1. True
The blood picture in chronic myeloid leukaemia is dominated by the presence of myelocytes, polymorphonuclear leucocytes and intermediate forms. In addition because the condition arises from the neoplastic transformation or clonal expansion of a pluripotential stem cell, basophils and eosinophils are also found in the peripheral blood.

2. False
The total white count is highest in chronic myeloid leukaemia reaching 300 000 per μl as compared to 100 000 per μl in the latter.

3. True
The Philadelphia chromosome is an abnormal 22 chromosome present in the white and red blood cell precursors in the marrow in chronic myeloid leukaemia.

4. False
Both diseases are commoner in middle and later life although chronic myeloid leukaemia occasionally occurs in younger individuals.

5. True
Many patients who have suffered from chronic myeloid leukaemia may enter a terminal phase in which acute leukaemia develops. This is associated with anaemia, infection and thrombocytopenic bleeding.

17.20 Chronic lymphatic leukaemia is associated with:
1. a marked increase in the number of lymphocytes in the peripheral blood
2. is not associated with hepatosplenomegaly
3. in some cases thrombocytopenia
4. an increase in the serum globulin concentration
5. chromosomal abnormalities

1. True
The number of white cells in the peripheral blood may reach 100 000 per ml. The majority of these are B lymphocytes with the appearance of normal mature small lymphocytes; only a small proportion are larger more primitive cells.

2. False
Generalized lymphadenopathy and hepatosplenomegaly are present in the majority of cases.

3. True
In about 15% of cases autoantibodies develop against red blood cells and platelets resulting in an autoimmune haemolytic anaemia and thrombocytopenia.

4. False
Because leukaemic B cells fail to respond to antigenic stimulation in CLL, a hypogammaglobulinaemia occurs together with an increased susceptibility to infection.

5. True
Approximately 50% of patients suffering from CLL have abnormal karyotypes, Trisomy 12 being the most common, seen in about one third of patients. This finding is indicative of a poor prognosis,

whereas abnormalities of 13q do not appear to affect the clinical course of the disease.

17.21 Monocytic leukaemia, now more commonly known as hairy cell leukaemia:
1. is the commonest form of leukaemia
2. is associated with monocytes or monoblasts in the peripheral blood
3. may present with increasing anaemia
4. is associated with nodular infiltrative skin lesions
5. can present as an acute myelo-monocytic form

1. False
Monocytic leukaemia is a relatively uncommon form of leukaemia. It accounts for less than 10% of all the leukaemias although it accounts for approximately 20% of acute leukaemias

2. True
The total white count may be relatively low although it may reach 250 000 per μl, the majority of cells being monocytes or monoblasts. These may exhibit pseudopodial cytoplasmic projections, a fine peripheral cytoplasmic PAS+ve granularity and lysozyme production.

3. True
This is a characteristic feature, however, of all types of leukaemia. Severe anaemia may arise so suddenly that the individual is prostrated with weakness.

4. True
This is one of the characteristic features of this type of leukaemia, the skin being infiltrated by monocytes or monoblasts.

5. True
This is the Naegeli type of leukaemia in which an admixture of myeloid cells and monoblasts appears, presumably due to the progenitor cell being able to differentiate into either type of cell line.

17.22 An enlarged lymph node which is excised is found by histological examination to be packed with tubercles consisting of epithelioid cells and giant cells. The tuberculin and Heaf tests are negative. Which of the following diseases should then be considered as the probable cause of the lymphadenopathy:
1. Hodgkin's disease
2. tuberculosis
3. sarcoidosis
4. syphilis
5. toxoplasmosis

1. False

Hodgkin's disease is not associated with follicle formation or epithelioid cells although giant cells, known as Reed–Sternberg cells, do appear.

2. False

If the node was tuberculous either the tuberculin or Heaf test should be positive.

3. True

This the classic picture of a node affected by sarcoidosis. The giant cells of sarcoidosis resemble foreign body giant cells rather than the Langhans cells characteristic of tuberculosis. A further pathological difference is that caseation does not occur in the centre of the follicles. The diagnosis can be confirmed by the presence of a positive Kveim Test.

4. False

In 'secondary syphilis' a generalized enlargement of the lymph nodes occurs some 2 to 3 months after exposure. Affected nodes show an increased number of plasma cells and macrophages and specific investigations such as the Wassermann reaction would be necessary to confirm the diagnosis.

5. False

The chief histological features of lymph nodes affected by toxoplasmosis are the presence of large cells, probably macrophages, scattered singly or in small groups throughout both the cortex and medulla. The sinuses are filled with smaller cells of uncertain nature. Toxoplasmosis is due to infection with the protozoon, *Toxoplasma gondii*.

17.23 Hodgkin's lymphoma has recently been reclassified into four histological groups. Regardless of classification, however, which of the following cell types are found in the lymph nodes in this disease:
1. lymphocytes
2. basophils
3. eosinophils
4. Reed–Sternberg cells
5. polymorphonuclear leucocytes

1. True

In all forms of Hodgkin's disease these cells are found in the lymph nodes. They are, however, most commonly found in the lymphocytic predominant type of the disease (Rye Classification).

2. False

Basophilic white cells are not found in the lymph nodes in any type of Hodgkin's disease.

3. True
Eosinophils are found particularly in the lymphocyte predominant and the nodular sclerotic types (Rye Classification).

4. True
These cells were described by Reed in 1902 and by Sternberg in 1898 and are usually known as Reed–Sternberg cells despite the fact that the same cell had already been described some years previously by Greenfield of Edinburgh in 1878. The Reed–Sternberg cell is a giant cell in which the nucleus is bifid or bilobed, the two halves being virtually identical. When more than two nuclei are present they are usually arranged in a horse shoe fashion or piled one on top of another. These are the typical cells of Hodgkin's disease and are present in all varieties of the disease although most common in 'mixed cellularity' type of disease.

5. True
Polymorphonuclear leucocytes are found either diffusely infiltrating affected lymph nodes or in marked aggregations suggesting the presence of micro-abscesses in the nodes.

17.24 The chief characteristics of Burkitt's lymphoma are:
1. that it is most common in young adults
2. it is associated with the Epstein–Barr virus
3. it is uncommon in malarial areas
4. the most common parts of the body involved are the facial bones and lower jaw
5. the characteristic cells of the tumour are poorly differentiated large lymphocytes and large pale histiocytes

1. False
This condition affects children in East and Central Africa but sporadic cases occur throughout the world.

2. True
This virus has been implicated in four types of human tumours, the African form of Burkitt's lymphoma, B-cell lymphomas in immunocompromised individuals, some cases of Hodgkin's lymphoma and nasopharyngeal carcinoma. In man 90% of African Burkitt's, the EB virus genome can be found in the B cell and 100% of patients have elevated antibody titres against the viral capsid antigens. Human EBV infection is not limited to areas in which Burkitt's lymphomas are found. It is known to cause infectious mononucleosis which is a self healing disease. It appears therefore that it is merely one factor involved in the development of Burkitt's lymphoma.

3. False
The most common areas in which the disease is found are the malarial areas although it occasionally occurs elsewhere. This association with malaria suggests that an infective oncogenic agent transmitted by insects plays a role in the aetiology.

4. True

In approximately 50% of all cases either the upper or lower jaws are involved and the teeth become loosened as the bones expand. Other regions involved are the lymph nodes of the abdomen, although the liver and spleen are rarely diseased.

5. True

The characteristic histological appearance of a Burkitt's lymphoma is a field of lymphocytes between 10–25 μm in diameter with a moderate amount of faintly basophilic or amphophilic cytoplasm. A high mitotic index is present and also a large number of dead cells, the latter accounting for the presence of numerous mononuclear phagocytes containing ingested nuclear debris. Randomly and diffusely distributed, the macrophages, often surrounded by a clear space, give rise to the descriptive term—'starry sky pattern'.

17.25 The plasma prothrombin time is increased:

1. in hepatocellular disease
2. in obstructive jaundice
3. in haemophilia
4. in Christmas disease
5. following splenectomy

1. True

Severe hepatocellular disease is incompatible with the normal synthesis of prothrombin and as a result the prothrombin time is prolonged.

2. True

In obstructive jaundice a decrease in prothrombin concentration occurs because obstruction of the biliary tree prevents bile salts entering the gut. As a result the fat soluble vitamin K, which is essential for prothrombin formation, fails to be absorbed.

3. False

The disease, although associated with bleeding, is due to the absence of the procoagulant activity of Factor VIII. The prothrombin time is normal.

4. False

This condition, first recognised in 1952, is due to a congenital absence of Factor IX. The prothrombin time is normal.

5. False

Splenectomy does not affect the prothrombin time but may be associated with a temporary thrombocythaemia. This may cause post-operative thrombotic episodes to occur.

17.26 Disorder of clotting occur in association with:

1. vitamin A deficiency
2. vitamin K deficiency

3. hereditary angioneurotic oedema
4. haemophilia
5. obstructive jaundice

1. False
Vitamin A plays no part in the clotting mechanisms but is concerned with the maintenance of the normal structure and function of epithelial tissues. Avitaminosis A results in squamous metaplasia in a number of epithelial tissues and in addition night blindness due to a deficiency of rhodopsin pigment in the retina.

2. True
Vitamin K is necessary for the hepatic synthesis of prothrombin and clotting factors VII, IX and X. Because of this the prothrombin time is increased in the presence of a vitamin K deficiency. Vitamin K deficiency accompanies many of the malabsorption syndromes.

3. False
Hereditary angioneurotic oedema is due to the absence of Cl esterase inhibitor which inhibits the action of Hageman factor. This defect causes an increase in the amount of kallikrein and an increased production of kinin. No direct effect on the clotting cascade occurs.

4. True
Haemophilia is a hereditary condition due to a sex linked recessive deficiency of antihaemophilic globulin or clotting Factor VIII. This results in a severe bleeding diathesis, bleeding being most commonly precipitated by trauma and involving the muscles and joints rather than the mucous membranes and the skin.

5. True
Both vitamin K deficiency and hypoprothrombinaemia occur in obstructive jaundice due to the exclusion of bile salts from the intestine which results in an inability to absorb fat soluble vitamins.

17.27 The formation of a clot is affected by the following substances:
1. zinc
2. calcium
3. Factor B
4. Factor IX
5. kallikrein

1. False
Zinc plays no role in clotting but is probably of some importance in wound healing.

2. True
Calcium ions are necessary for all phases of the clotting cascade.

3. False
Factor B plays no part in the clotting of blood. Factor B or C3

proactivator plays an important role in the alternative pathway of complement activation.

4. True
Factor IX or Christmas factor is part of the intrinsic clotting pathway. Deficiency of Factor IX occurs as a rare sex linked recessive trait producing a bleeding disorder similar to haemophilia.

5. False
Kallikrein is a part of the kinin system which generates mediators such as bradykinin and lysyl-bradykinin or kallidin. Bradykinin is a powerful vasoactive nonapeptide which causes vasodilatation and increased vascular permeability. It is one of the many mediators of the inflammatory response.

17.28 Haemorrhagic lesions may occur as a result of:
1. vitamin B deficiency
2. vitamin C deficiency
3. retinol deficiency
4. the nephrotic syndrome
5. penicillin therapy

1. False
Vitamin B deficiency is not associated with haemorhagic lesions. Classically thiamine deficiency causes bori-beri; riboflavine deficiency, angular stomatitis and glossitis and nicotinic acid deficiency pellagra which is associated with dermatitis, diarrhoea and dementia.

2. True
Vitamin C (ascorbic acid) is important in the production of collagen and in the synthesis of intercellular cement of the vascular endothelium. Avitaminosis C causes one of the classical deficiency diseases, i.e. scurvy, one of the manifestations of which is the appearance of haemorrhagic lesions particularly involving the gums and skin around the base of the hair follicles.

3. False
Retinol is vitamin A; deficiency of this vitamin does not cause haemorrhagic lesions. It causes night blindness followed by xerophthalmia and keratomalacia.

4. False
There is no tendency to develop haemorrhagic lesions in the nephrotic syndrome which is associated with widespread subcutaneous oedema due to loss of protein in the urine.

5. True
Procaine penicillin is one of a group of drugs including aspirin, phenacetin and the sulphonamides which may give rise to petechial haemorrhages in the skin. The basis of the phenomenon may be an immune complex related to the Arthus phenomenon and in a number of other situations including aspirin idiosyncrasy, an allergic reaction cannot be excluded.

17.29 Disseminated intravascular coagulation occurs as a complication of:
1. many obstetrical complications
2. malignant disease
3. polycythaemia vera
4. the overadministration of thrombokinase
5. endotoxaemic shock

1. True
Abruptio placenta, septic abortion, amniotic fluid embolisation and toxaemia of pregnancy may all be followed by DIC, due to the liberation of thromboplastins which trigger the extrinsic pathway with the additional factor that widespread endothelial damage also occurs.

2. True
Patients suffering from malignant disease of the prostate, bronchus, pancreas and stomach are particularly liable to this complication due to the liberation of thromboplastins.

3. False
Polycythaemia vera is a condition usually seen in middle age. The basic pathological change is in the bone marrow which is markedly hypercellular, the fatty marrow being replaced by haemopoetic red marrow as the condition progresses. As a result of the erythrocytosis, there is an increase in blood volume and blood viscosity and as a result of the latter vascular stasis, thromboses and infarctions occur. The presence of an absolute polycythaemia is confirmed by demonstrating that a patient's red cell mass exceeds 40 ml/kg. The condition, although complicated by venous thromboses, is not normally associated with DIC.

4. False
Thrombokinase is used in the treatment of patients in whom intravascular thrombosis and coagulation has occurred. It has been used for example in patients who have suffered from a pulmonary embolus.

5. True
Gram-negative infections, by releasing endotoxins, may activate both the intrinsic and extrinsic pathways by producing endothelial cell damage and the release of thromboplastins from inflammatory cells. In addition, endotoxins inhibit the anticoagulant activity of protein C by suppressing thrombomodulin expression on endothelium and also are capable of directly activating Factor XII.

17.30 The following functions are carried out by platelets:
1. binding of antigen-antibody complexes
2. secretion of clotting factors
3. secretion of prostaglandins

4. release of the Hageman factor
5. release of vasoactive amines

1. True
Antigen-antibody complexes activate complement and are bound to platelets by a process known as immune adherence through a receptor for C3b.

2. False
Although platelets play a vital role in haemostasis they do not release any of the factors concerned in either the intrinsic or extrinsic clotting pathways. Plasma contains all the factors necessary for clotting to take place after contact activation or tissue damage. Platelet factor 3 is an altered state of the surface of the platelets and not a secretion.

3. True
Platelets release prostaglandin E_2. This is concerned with the release of ADP, a substance which causes the platelets to adhere together. E type prostaglandins are also proinflammatory agents, acting via cyclic AMP.

4. False
The Hageman factor (Factor XII) is a plasma protein which migrates on electrophoresis as a β or γ globulin. It is activated by contact and this is the first step in the intrinsic clotting pathway.

5. True
Platelets release 5-hydroxytryptamine (serotonin) which is a potent vasoactive material causing vasodilatation and an increase in capillary permeability.

17.31 Thrombocytopenia can be caused by:
1. deficiency of clotting factors
2. haemorrhage
3. diuretics
4. measles virus
5. telangiectasia

1. False
A deficiency of clotting factors causes bleeding diseases such as haemophilia and Christmas disease, but there is no reduction in platelet numbers in either of these conditions. Thrombocytopenia is, however, associated with a bleeding diathesis, because platelets are necessary for haemostasis. Platelets seal small vessels, which are injured, by adhering to their surface, catalysing the intrinsic clotting system through surface lipoprotein.

2. True
Severe haemorrhage or repeated bleeding may cause thrombocytopenia. This loss, if severe, must be made good by the transfusion of fresh blood. Stored blood does not contain viable platelets and is, therefore, useless.

3. True

The thiazide diuretics are among the many drugs which can give rise to a thrombocytopenia. This is considered to be produced immunologically by the binding of the drug to the platelets. Antibody is then being formed against the drug which acts as a hapten.

4. True

Viruses, such as the measles virus, may impair platelet production by colonising the parent megakaryocytes. Others may actually destroy platelets or form immune complexes binding to the platelets leading to their destruction.

5. False

Hereditary haemorrhagic telangiectasia may be the cause of haemorrhages due to the associated vascular defect even though the concentration of clotting factors and the number of platelets is normal.

17.32 Thrombocytopenia:
1. may occur as an autoimmune phenomenon
2. is caused by sulphonamides
3. is associated with an increased bleeding time
4. is associated with an increased clotting time
5. the thromboplastin generation test is useful in its recognition

1. True

Idiopathic thrombocytopenic purpura is associated with IgG autoantibodies against platelets. A similar type of thrombocytopenia may occur in other recognised autoimmune diseases such as systemic lupus erythematosus. The accelerated removal of platelets from the circulation is primarily mediated by the splenic macrophages via the immune adherence receptors of these cells. In SLE autoantibodies to cardiolipin and other phospholipids may occasionally be detected.

2. True

Sulphonamides, thiazide diuretics, quinidine and stibophen, are among the drugs that give rise to thrombocytopenia. The drug that has been most extensively investigated is sedormid. In sedormid purpura this drug acts as a hapten, which binds to the serum proteins with the result that antibody formation occurs. Antigen-antibody complexes then bind to the platelets resulting in their destruction.

3. True

The bleeding time, normally between 1 and 9 minutes, is the time taken for a small puncture to stop bleeding. The duration of the bleeding time is dependent upon normal platelet activity and thrombocytopenia, therefore, from whatever cause, will cause a prolonged bleeding time.

4. False
This is the time taken for blood to clot in a test tube and normally takes between 5 and 15 minutes. An increase in the clotting time occurs when there is a deficiency of clotting factors as in haemophilia whereas in thrombocytopenia the clotting time is normal.

5. False
The thromboplastin generation test is a complex test which is used to identify particular defects in the clotting factors in the serum. In the first stage thromboplastin (prothrombinase) is generated using a mixture of serum, kaolin absorbed plasma, platelets and calcium. The thromboplastin is then assayed by adding the mixture to normal plasma. This test will not help in the diagnosis of thrombocytopenia, although it is extremely valuable in pointing to the precise defect in the clotting factors.

17.33 Platelets contribute to haemostasis by liberating:
1. 5-hydroxytryptamine (serotonin)
2. phospholipids
3. plasminogen
4. bradykinin
5. calcitonin

1. True
5-hydroxytryptamine liberated from the platelets is a vasoconstrictor augmenting the normal vascular contraction which follows injury.

2. True
Platelet phospholipid and calcium is essential to the intrinsic coagulation system.

3. False
Plasminogen is the inactive precursor of plasmin which is carried in the plasma. Whenever fibrinogen is laid down it carries with it sufficient plasminogen to ensure its subsequent lysis.

4. False
Bradykinin is a powerful vasodilator probably derived from an α_2-globulin in the plasma by the action of the enzyme kallikrein.

5. False
This hormone is derived from the parafollicular (C) cells of the thyroid and is one of three important factors concerned in the regulation of plasma calcium concentration, the other factors being parathyroid hormone and vitamin D_3. It has no effect on haemostasis.

17.34 Thrombocytopenic purpura differs from non-thrombocytopenic purpura in that:
1. in the former condition the platelet count is reduced
2. in the latter the main defect is in the capillaries

3. the former may follow systemic disease
4. the latter may result from allergy
5. petechiae occur in the former but not in the latter

1. True
When the platelet count is reduced below 150 000 per µl thrombocytopenia is present. Abnormal bleeding is uncommon, however, if the platelet count remains higher than 60 000 per µl.

2. True
Platelets are normally involved in preventing bleeding from capillaries. When the platelet count is normal but the capillaries are abnormal, e.g. due to the action of endotoxins, bleeding occurs.

3. True
Among the many causes of thrombocytopenic purpura are systemic lupus erythematosus and chronic lymphatic leukaemia.

4. True
The classical example of non-thrombocytopenic purpura is Henoch–Schönlein purpura, otherwise known as anaphylactoid purpura. This condition commonly develops some 2 to 3 weeks after a streptococcal upper respiratory infection.

5. False
In both types of purpura small haemorrhages occur from capillaries throughout the body causing petechiae in the skin, mucous membranes and serous surfaces. Bleeding into the mucous membrane of the gastrointestinal tract produces abdominal colic, bleeding in the urinary tract produces haematuria.

17.35 Consecutive clot:
1. occurs in arteries distal to a thrombotic obstruction
2. occurs in the collateral branches of an artery following obstruction to the main vessel
3. occurs in veins after the cessation of blood flow
4. extends proximally to the entrance of the next venous tributary
5. is formed of coralline thrombus

1. False
Consecutive clot occurs only in veins.

2. False
For the above reason.

3. True
When the blood flow in a vein has come to a halt the process of thrombosis begins and clotting follows. A consecutive clot develops proximal to that point at which stagnation becomes complete. Normally the clot extends proximally to the entrance of the next venous tributary. At this point the tip of the clot may become invaded by granulation tissue from the wall of the vessel in which the clot is

occurring and its surface may become covered with endothelium. By this means propagation of the clot is halted. Alternatively clotting may continue proximally over a considerable distance leading to the clinical syndromes of phlegmasia alba or caerulea dolens.

4. True
As stated above

5. False
Coralline thrombus occurs in veins in which the blood is still flowing. This type of thrombus is so named because it is composed of alternating layers of fused platelets and fibrin, the latter containing entrapped red cells. This configuration is best seen on longitudinal sections through the centre of the thrombus. Retraction of the fibrin causes a ripple effect and the elevated platelet ridges between the fibrin form the so-called lines of Zahn.

SECTION 18. ENDOCRINOLOGY

18.1 Phaeochromocytoma may be associated with:
1. paroxysmal hypertension
2. sweating
3. neurofibromatosis
4. a fall in blood pressure on palpating the abdomen
5. paroxysmal hypotension

1. True
Paroxysmal hypertension usually occurs early in the disease when noradrenaline is being intermittently released. Commonly, however, by the time a clinical diagnosis is reached a sustained hypertension is present due to constant outpouring of catechol amines.

2. True
This symptom, also due to the overproduction of catechol amines, may be paroxysmal or continuous.

3. True
Neurofibromatosis occurs in association with phaeochromocytoma in 5% of all patients.

4. False
In approximately 50% of patients suffering from phaeochromocytoma palpating the abdomen on the side of the tumour leads to a rise in blood pressure.

5. True
The possible explanation for this phenomenon is that an increase in the concentration of circulating catechol amines leads to a decrease in plasma and total blood volume.

18.2 Increased amounts of erythropoietin are found in the plasma:
1. in pernicious anaemia
2. in iron deficiency anaemia
3. following bleeding
4. in erythroblastosis fetalis
5. in kwashiorkor

1. True
2. True
3. True
4. True
5. False

Erythropoietin is a lineage specific cytokine specifically stimulating the production of red cells. A similar factor, macrophage colony stimulating factor (M-CSF) stimulates the production of macrophages. It is a glycoprotein which can be inactivated by mild acid hydrolysis or by inducing the formation of antibodies. Its production is regulated by an exquisitely sensitive feed back mechanism and in man only a relatively minor bleed is necessary to produce a rapid increase in the plasma concentration.

Erythropoietin may be formed in the kidney. An alternative hypothesis has, however, been advanced suggesting that the kidney produces a renal erythropoietin factor (REF). This then behaves like an enzyme acting upon a substrate in the plasma.

Increased amounts are found in the plasma in all conditions listed above with the exception of kwashiorkor.

18.3 An eosinophil adenoma of the anterior hypophysis is associated with:
1. enlargement of the sella turcica
2. hypertrophy and hyperplasia of the soft tissues throughout the body
3. excessive growth of the acral parts
4. premature closure of the epiphyses
5. impaired glucose tolerance

1. True
Eosinophil adenomata commonly grow to such a size that the sella turcica is enlarged, this being usually demonstrated by radiological examination. In addition enlargement of the gland causes pressure on the optic chiasma which eventually causes visual impairment in over half the cases.

2. True
Hyperplasia and hypertrophy occur because the secretion of somatotrophin (growth hormone) is excessive in this type of tumour. Should, however, the tumour undergo cystic degeneration or infarction the progressive development of gigantism or acromegaly ceases.

3. True
This is the change which gives rise to the name 'acromegaly'. Acromegaly occurs when the excessive somatotrophin excretion begins following fusion of the epiphyses and, therefore, only about 40% of acromegalic patients gain in height. In the majority of sufferers the hands become 'spade-like' due to an overgrowth of the soft tissues and cortical thickening of the phalangeal bones, together with 'tufting' of the distal phalanges.

4. False
Fusion of the epiphyses occurs normally. However, the time at which somatotrophin overproduction begins is important. If oversecretion begins prior to fusion of the epiphyses gigantism develops with the long bones participating in proportionate growth whereas if oversecretion begins after epiphyseal fusion little increase in height normally occurs and the classic acromegalic is produced.

5. True
Impaired glucose tolerance occurs in about 50% of patients and clinical diabetes in about 10%.

18.4   Primary thyrotoxicosis is always accompanied by:
1. increased iodine uptake by the gland
2. a raised protein bound iodine
3. exophthalmos
4. hypercalcaemia
5. pernicious anaemia

1. True
Except in T_3 thyrotoxicosis hyperthyroidism is almost invariably associated with an increased uptake of iodine. Uptake is also increased in disorders in which accumulated iodine is inefficiently or ineffectively used to synthesize and secrete active hormone and in conditions in which there is excessive hormone losses as in nephrosis, in which there is excessive loss of hormone in the urine in association with the urinary loss of binding proteins.

2. True
This test was once the mainstay of thyroid diagnosis but is now seldom used. The serum PBI measures the following:
  (a) The iodine in T_4
  (b) The small quantities of iodine in T_3
  (c) A great variety of iodinated materials of exogenous origin that are bound to protein and a class of compounds, usually of endogenous origin, termed iodoproteins in which iodine is covalently bound within the peptide sequence of the protein molecule. The latter are commonly found in the sera of patients with Hashimoto's disease.

3. False
Exophthalmos is not necessarily present in patients suffering from

primary thyrotoxicosis. The mechanism by which exophthalmos is produced remains to be elucidated. There is no doubt, however, that the anatomical deformity is caused by the deposition of mucopolysaccharides in the retro-orbital fat and the extrinsic muscles of the eye. In the majority of patients suffering from exophthalmos the plasma contains raised levels of LATS which is a gamma-globulin distinct from TSH.

4. True
Thyrotoxicosis is associated with increased excretion of calcium and phosphorus in the urine and stool. In some patients this may be so great that bone density is reduced and pathological fractures occur.

5. False
Approximately 3% of patients with primary thyrotoxicosis have pernicious anaemia and a further 3% have intrinsic factor autoantibody together with a normal absorption of vitamin B_{12}.

18.5 Abnormal aggregation of lymphocytes occurs in the thyroid in the following pathological conditions:
1. follicular carcinoma
2. medullary carcinoma
3. lymphadenoid goitre
4. Reidel's struma
5. primary thyrotoxicosis

1. False
An excessive lymphocytic infiltration does not occur in this condition which is one of the two well differentiated forms of malignant disease of the thyroid. Some areas of such a tumour bear a close resemblance to normal thyroid tissue although the follicles generally are smaller and contain lesser amounts of colloid but in other areas the tumour is composed of solid sheets of cells.

2. False
Medullary tumours comprise only 5 to 10% of thyroid neoplasms. They consist of cells with widely varying morphological features and arrangements in which papillary folds or follicles do not occur. An abundant hyaline stroma is present which has the staining properties of amyloid.

3. True
Lymphocytic infiltration is the characteristic feature of lymphadenoid goitre (Hashimoto's disease). In the majority of cases histological examination of the gland also reveals the destruction of the follicular cells and degeneration and fragmentation of the surrounding basement membrane. The interstitial tissue is infiltrated with lymphocytes, plasma cells, immunoblasts, and macrophages and typical lymphoid follicles with germinal centres may be seen.

4. False
In Reidel's thyroiditis the thyroid undergoes a fibrotic change which extends into the adjacent structures. This change may be associated with abnormal fibrosis elsewhere in the body especially in the posterior mediastinum, producing superior mediastinal obstruction and in the retroperitoneal tissues causing the development of bilateral hydronephrosis and eventually renal failure.

5. True
The characteristic histopathological picture of primary thyrotoxicosis is one in which the follicles are small and lined by hyperplastic columnar epithelium with in addition varying degrees of lymphocytic infiltration which may form lymphoid follicles.

18.6   Primary hyperparathyroidism is associated with:
1. bone cysts
2. carcinoma of the parathyroid glands
3. dystrophic calcification
4. hypertension
5. anorexia

1. True
Histological examination of the bones in primary hyperparathyroidism shows generalized osteitis fibrosa. An increased formation and resorption of bone is evident and excessive numbers of osteoclasts can be seen on the trabeculae. The underlying cause of the osseous manifestations of hyperparathyroidism is the hypersecretion of parathyroid hormone which, detected by receptors on the osteoblasts, initiates the release of mediators which stimulates osteoblastic activity.

2. True
Carcinoma is the rarest parathyroid pathology causing primary hyperparathyroidism, a malignant tumour of a solitary gland accounting for only approximately 2% of all cases. Clinically, malignancy should be suspected if a mass is palpable in the neck.

3. False
Dystrophic classification only occurs in degenerate tissues. In primary hyperparathyroidism the accompanying hypercalcaemia is followed by metastatic calcification in normal tissues such as the kidney causing nephrocalcinosis. Calcium deposits develop in the cytoplasm and on the basement membrane of the tubular epithelial cells. Calcified cellular debris then causes obstruction of the tubular lumina causing obstructive atrophy of the nephrons with interstitial fibrosis and a non-specific chronic inflammation. Renal functional defects which can be demonstrated include: tubular acidosis, salt losing nephritis and finally renal failure.

4. True
Hypertension occurs in primary hyperparathyroidism when the

degree of renal damage produced by the development of nephrocalcinosis has become severe enough to impair renal function.

5. True
The anorexia accompanying primary hyperparathyroidism may be due to one of three causes:
(a) The hypercalcaemia alone
(b) The presence of a co-existing duodenal ulcer
(c) Recurrent pancreatitis

18.7 The plasma acid phosphatase concentration increases in:
1. Paget's disease (osteitis deformans)
2. idiopathic hypercalciuria
3. prostatic cancer
4. medullary carcinoma of the thyroid
5. rickets

1. False
Osteitis deformans is associated with an elevation of the alkaline phosphatase, the acid phosphatase is unaffected.

2. False
Idiopathic hypercalciuria is not associated with any change in the acid phosphatase levels. The high renal calcium output in this condition is possibly caused by the excessive intestinal absorption of this cation by an increase in vitamin-D-like or $1,25 (OH)_2 D_3$ activity.

3. True
In prostatic cancer the acid phosphatase rises above the normal level of 0 to 4 KA units/100 ml. High values occur particularly when the disease is disseminated because both normal and malignant prostatic epithelium secrete large quantities of this enzyme.

4. False
The only significant biochemical abnormality associated with medullary tumours of the thyroid is the hypersecretion of calcitonin.

5. False
Classical rickets is caused by a deficient intake of vitamin D in infancy. An increase in the concentration of alkaline phosphatase occurs without any change in the acid phosphatase.

18.8 The Zollinger–Ellison syndrome is associated with:
1. β-cell tumours of the pancreas
2. chronic duodenal ulceration
3. cholereiform diarrhoea
4. parathyroid adenomata
5. phaeochromocytoma

1. False
This syndrome is caused by non-β-cell islet cell tumours which in approximately two thirds of patients are malignant. This is clinically important since the surgeon may be forced to direct his attention to the target organ, i.e. the stomach, leaving the tumour itself *in situ*.

2. True
The stomach is maximally stimulated by the presence of the gastrin secreting tumour and chronic duodenal ulceration follows. These ulcers may be multiple and even occur in the descending part of the duodenum or upper jejunum.

3. True
The gastric acid is normally neutralized by the alkaline pancreatic juices but the large quantities of acid secreted in this syndrome cannot be neutralized by this means. Thus excessive quantities of acid reach the small bowel causing an acid enteritis associated with exceedingly fluid stools. An additional factor is probably the direct hormonal effect of gastrin on the transport of fluid and electrolytes.

4. True
Islet cell tumours producing gastrin are sometimes associated with parathyroid and pituitary adenomata. This particular 'cluster' is known as multiple endocrine adenoma, Type I.

5. False
Phaeochromocytoma are not associated with the Zollinger–Ellison syndrome but with medullary carcinoma of the thyroid and less frequently parathyroid adenomata, the MEN 11a syndrome.

18.9 The following tumours of the ovary secrete hormones:
1. arrhenoblastoma
2. dysgerminoma
3. dermoid cysts
4. papillary cystadenoma
5. granulosa-theca cell tumour

1. True
These tumours which account for less than 1% of all solid ovarian tumours secrete androgens with the result that masculinisation takes place in affected women. Around 70% occur below the age of forty.

2. False
These tumours are the ovarian counterpart of seminoma of the testes. They account for only about 2% of all malignant ovarian tumours and are commonest between 10–30 years of age. The majority have no endocrine function but a few secrete chorionic gonadotrophins.

3. True
Dermoid cysts may contain foci of chromaffin tissue which secrete serotonin. Rarer still are cysts consisting almost exclusively of thyroid tissue, the struma ovarii, which are sufficiently differentiated to produce thyroxine causing thyrotoxicosis.

4. False
Papillary cystadenoma is one of the commoner tumours of the ovary. They are frequently bilateral, commonly reaching 10 cm in diameter. They may consist of a single main cyst on the inner surface of which are multiple papilliform projections. The contents are usually clear fluid unless complications such as torsion have occurred.

5. True
This tumour accounts for between 15 and 20% of all solid ovarian neoplasms. Producing oestrogens they commonly present with polymenorrhoea but they may also produce androgens and so cause virilism with associated hirsutism and increasing libido.

18.10 Diabetes insipidus is associated with:
1. the oversecretion of vasopressin
2. polydipsia
3. a urine specific gravity greater than 1020
4. head injury
5. metastatic cancer

1. False
The cause of diabetes insipidus is a deficiency of vasopressin. This causes the uncontrollable diuresis which leads to the accompanying polyuria. Vasopressin alters the responsiveness of the plasma membrane on the luminal surface of the tubular cells.

2. True
The polyuria of diabetes insipidus is accompanied by polydipsia. Increasing thirst leads to a grossly increased intake of water.

3. False
The urine specific gravity in diabetes insipidus rarely rises above 1005.

4. True
A head injury which results in damage to the hypothalamus may result in diabetes insipidus. However, neither destruction of the neurohypophysis nor high transection of the pituitary stalk usually cause diabetes insipidus because sufficient ADH escapes from the severed neurohypophyseal tract.

5. True
If metastatic cancer involves the hypothalamus diabetes insipidus may follow.

SECTION 19. THE RENAL SYSTEM

19.1 Renal function is depressed in the following conditions:
1. 'shock'
2. amyloidosis
3. chronic hyperuricaemia
4. irradiation
5. hypercalcaemia

1. True
'Shock', particularly when due to loss of water and salt or haemorrhage, depresses renal function by causing severe renal vasoconstriction. Following severe blood loss, if the blood volume remains reduced for several hours, the renal vasoconstriction may be sufficiently severe to cause tubular or glomerular necrosis. Fortunately the former is more common and is reversible.

2. True
Amyloidosis, which follows chronic sepsis or rheumatoid arthritis, may also occur as a familial condition. When the kidney is affected proteinuria follows and the nephrotic syndrome develops. Occasionally renal vein thrombosis occurs to produce acute renal failure.

3. True
Chronic hyperuricaemia causes chronic renal failure by the production of interstitial nephritis, nephrosclerosis and possibly the development of uric acid stones.

4. True
If the kidneys are not protected from irradiation, for example, during the treatment of malignant para-aortic glands, they will be damaged. The onset of symptoms often follows a latent interval of 6 to 12 months after which oedema, dyspnoea, hypertension, headache, nausea and vomiting, lassitude and nocturia occur. Death usually occurs due to hypertensive cardiac failure, hypertensive fits and renal failure.

5. True
Hypercalcaemia leads to hypercalciuria which in turn leads to nephrocalcinosis. At this stage renal function is depressed due to the tubular defect which is produced.

19.2 The renal control of acid base balance is a function of the:
1. loop of Henlé
2. proximal tubule
3. glomerulus
4. distal tubule
5. collecting tubule

1. False
2. False

3. **False**
4. **True**
5. **False**

Acids in the body are taken up by buffer system:

$$H^+A + NaHCO_3 \rightleftharpoons Na A + H_2CO_3 \rightleftharpoons H_2O + CO_2$$
(acid produced by some
metabolic process)

The carbon dioxide is excreted by the lungs and the anion by the kidney but if this was excreted together with the sodium ion, the net result of the production of one hydrogen ion would be the loss from the body of one molecule of sodium bicarbonate. This depletion is prevented by the formation of carbonic acid within the cells of the distal tubules under the control of carbonic anhydrase. The cell then exchanges hydrogen for sodium in the tubular lumen and sodium bicarbonate is returned to the blood. A further mechanism involved is the production of ammonia by the cells of the distal tubule. The ammonia ion combines with a hydrogen ion and a chloride ion in the tubular lumen, sodium is reabsorbed in the exchange and ammonium chloride is excreted in the urine.

19.3 **In renal tubular acidosis the following biochemical abnormalities occur:**
1. an inability to lower the urine pH
2. abnormal ammonia excretion in relation to urine pH
3. renal glycosuria
4. hypercalciuria
5. hyperkalaemia

1. True
The inability to lower urine pH is due to an inability to produce and maintain a hydrogen ion gradient between the tubule lumen and the cell. With normal quantities of buffer in the urine the impaired ability to lower the urine pH results in a reduced excretion of titratable acid.

2. False
Ammonia excretion is usually normal in relation to the urine pH, but as the urine pH cannot be reduced the absolute excretion of ammonia is nearly always low.

3. False
Renal glycosuria does not occur.

4. True
Hypercalciuria can occur and may be associated with nephrocalcinosis although they may occur independently. The hypercalciuria is due to the systemic acidosis because the hydrogen ions tend to be buffered by bone with the release of calcium into extracellular fluid.

5. False
Increased potassium excretion occurs leading to hypokalaemia. This is due to systemic acidosis and also secondary aldosteronism which develops when the affected patients become sodium depleted.

19.4 The nephrotic syndrome is accompanied by:
1. decreased glomerular capillary permeability
2. oedema
3. a loss of 10 g or more of plasma protein daily
4. hypolipidaemia
5. abundant cortical deposits of neutral fat and anisotropic lipids.

1. False
The major defect in the nephrotic syndrome is an increase in glomerular capillary permeability. This may occur in various types of glomerulonephritis, e.g. membranoproliferative glomerulonephritis which most commonly occurs in older children.

2. True
Generalized oedema occurs chiefly due to the loss of colloid osmotic pressure caused by the heavy proteinuria. An additional factor is sodium and water retention which is caused by the compensatory secretion of aldosterone mediated by the enhanced secretion of antidiuretic hormone and a reduction in the secretion of atrial peptides. It should be remembered that conditions other than renal disease may produce the same effect, e.g. protein losing enteropathy and chronic malnutrition.

3. True
It is this huge loss of albumin which leads to the associated generalized oedema by reducing the osmotic pressure in the capillaries.

4. False
For reasons not understood the nephrotic syndrome is associated with hyperlipidaemia. Most patients have increased cholesterol, triglycerides, VLDL, LDL, but a decrease in high density lipoproteins HDL. These defects in part appear to be due to an increased synthesis of lipoproteins in the liver. Whereas in a normal individual the normal daily urinary excretion of fats is less than 10 mg, in the nephrotic syndrome this may rise to 1000 mg due to the hyperlipidaemia. The crystallisation of cholesterol esters gives rise to the classical birefringent urinary crystals.

5. True
The kidneys in the nephrotic syndrome are enlarged and pallid due to oedema and frequently a yellow, radial streaking of the cortex is present due to the deposition of lipids. Both anisotropic lipid and some sudanophil neutral fat (dark) is deposited in the interstitial tissue and tubules.

19.5 Acute tubular necrosis of the kidney commonly follows:
1. severe dehydration
2. the overadministration of carbon tetrachloride
3. acute porphyria
4. the overadministration of potassium chloride
5. gentamicin

1. True
Tubular necrosis follows severe dehydration because of the reduction in blood volume which results in renal ischaemia from two causes, first the reduced flow of blood through the kidney and secondly, the accompanying vasoconstriction. In this type of ATN short lengths of the tubules are affected involving both the descending and ascending loops of Henlé.

2. True
Carbon tetrachloride is a poison which acts directly on the tubular cells, along with many other poisons. The chief sites of necrosis include the proximal convoluted tubules and the descending loops of Henlé. In carbon tetrachloride poisoning, an accumulation of neutral lipids occurs in the injured cells.

3. True
Acute porphyria is often provoked by the administration of barbiturates. At autopsy large amounts of porphyrins can be identified in the tubule cells leading to tubular malfunction.

4. False
The potassium salt which causes renal damage is potassium chlorate. Potassium chloride administration is associated with mucosal ulceration of the small bowel leading to ulceration, possible perforation or stricture formation.

5. False
Both reversible nephrotoxicity and acute renal failure have been reported following the administration of gentamicin but they are rare. The chief danger associated with the administration of this antibiotic is vestibular damage and high tone hearing loss. This is particularly liable to occur in patients suffering from decreased renal function.

19.6 The differences between the tubular lesions produced by nephrotoxic drugs and renal ischaemia include:
1. the lesion produced by ischaemia occurs in a random fashion throughout all nephrons and in any part of the nephron down to collecting tubules
2. a nephrotoxic drug affects the entire nephron
3. nephrotoxic drugs produce scattered lesions throughout the kidney
4. ischaemia causes complete necrosis of the tubule cell together with the basement membrane
5. nephrotoxins cause both cytotoxic and ischaemic lesions

1. True

Ischaemic lesions of the kidney are associated with random lesions in which any part of the nephron may be affected.

2. False

Nephrotoxic drugs affect all nephrons equally and the lesions are confined to the same part of each proximal tubule.

3. False

The effect of nephrotoxic drugs is to produce a generalized lesion throughout the kidney.

4. True

Complete necrosis of the tubule cells and the basement membrane exposes the lumen of the tubule to the renal interstitial space.

5. True

Nephrotoxins can cause ischaemic lesions because the cytotoxic agents in high concentration cause intense renal vasoconstriction.

19.7   Uretero-colic anastomosis is followed by:

1   ascending pyelonephritis
2. absorption of ammonium salts
3. absorption of urea from the colon
4. metabolic alkalosis
5. hyperkalaemia

1. True

This operation is invariably followed by the reflux of faecal material up the ureters, causing severe renal infection.

2. True

Ammonium salts are absorbed in excess from the bowel because of the ammonia formed from the urine by the urea splitting bacteria in the colon.

3. True

The reabsorption of urea from the urine by the colon is sufficient, even in the absence of any change in renal function, to cause a rise in the blood urea. It can be distinguished from a rise in blood urea due to a true depression of glomerular filtration by estimating the plasma creatinine since the latter is not absorbed from the bowel.

4. False

Uretero-colic anastomosis is followed by the reabsorption of chloride to a greater extent than sodium ions. This, together with the reabsorption of hydrogen ions, tends to cause an acidosis strictly known as hyperchloraemic acidosis.

5. False

Following uretero-colic anastomosis an excessive loss of potassium occurs probably due to two causes:
  (a) Increased quantities of urinary potassium are delivered into the colon once pyelonephritis develops.
  (b) Excessive loss from the colon itself due to the large amount of colonic mucus which is excreted due to irritation of the wall of the bowel by urine.

19.8 Haemoglobinuria occurs:
1. in blackwater fever
2. following the excessive ingestion of beetroot
3. following extensive superficial burns.
4. in blood transfusion
5. in strenuous exercise

1. True

Blackwater fever is the name given to a complication of malignant tertian malaria. It usually occurs in patients who have been previously treated with antimalarial drugs, particularly quinine, either prophylactically or for recurrent attacks of malaria. Sudden and severe haemolysis occurs followed in some cases by acute renal failure.

2. False

The urine may become red following the eating of beetroot due to the excretion of red dye of vegetable origin.

3. False

Superficial burns are not associated with haemoglobinuria. However, extensive deep full thickness burns are followed by this condition because of the direct exposure of red cells to the effect of heat in their passage through the area exposed to the responsible agent. The morphology of the cells is so altered that they are subsequently sequestrated and prematurely destroyed, liberating haemoglobin into the circulation which is then passed in the urine.

4. False

Blood transfusion is not followed by haemoglobinuria unless the transfused blood belongs to the incorrect group. Such mismatched blood is immediately haemolysed, the plasma concentration of haemoglobin rises and there is fever, shivering, severe pains in the back, hypotension and haemoglobinuria.

5. True

Any normal person who undergoes sufficiently severe and prolonged strenuous exercise will develop haemoglobinuria and proteinuria. This has been shown in marathon runners. It is a benign condition and associated with no late sequelae.

SECTION 20. WATER AND ELECTROLYTE DISTURBANCE

20.1   The major differences between the plasma and the interstitial fluid are in:
1. the concentration of sodium
2. the concentration of calcium
3. the bicarbonate concentration
4. the protein content
5. the organic acid concentration

1. True
The concentration of sodium in the former is 153 mmol/l (mEq/l) and in the latter 143 mmol/l (mEq/l).

2. False
The concentration of calcium is the same in both.

3. False
The concentration of bicarbonate ion is the same and equal in both.

4. True
The protein content of the plasma is approximately eight times greater than in the interstitial fluid.

5. False
The concentration of organic acid is the same in both.

20.2   The percentage of total body water in any individual is influenced by:
1. the lean body mass
2. the activity of the adrenal cortex
3. an increased sodium content of the diet
4. thyroid activity
5. vomiting

1. True
The total body water in a normal individual is particularly related to lean body mass. Since the lean body mass is greater in the male but decreases with age in both sexes the percentage of body water is always greater in the male than the female at any age.

2. True
Cortical hyperplasia and benign or malignant cortical tumours lead to the secretion of abnormal quantities of cortisol causing the retention of sodium and water.

3. False
Excessive quantities of sodium in the diet are absorbed and then excreted by the kidney due to diminished tubular reabsorption.

4. True
Overactivity of the thyroid, i.e. thyrotoxicosis, leads to proximal

muscle wasting and hence loss of lean body mass. Indirectly, therefore, thyrotoxicosis must be associated with a reduction in the percentage of total body water. Underactivity of the thyroid, however, which is associated with myxoedema, is associated with an increase in the mucopolysaccharides of the ground substance.

5. True
Persistent vomiting cause a reduction in extracellular fluid and hence of the percentage of total body water.

20.3 The renin-angiotensin-aldosterone system regulates:
1. potassium balance
2. sodium balance
3. fluid volume
4. blood pressure
5. nitrogen balance

1. True
Aldosterone acts to promote K^+ loss at the same time stimulating Na^+ reabsorption by the Na^+-K^+ ion exchange transport system. As the plasma potassium falls, aldosterone secretion is accordingly reduced.

2. True
Because sodium depletion is followed by a contraction of the effective blood volume and a fall in the arterial pressure renal perfusion diminishes and as a result renin is secreted into the blood stream. Renin then acts enzymatically on a plasma globulin causing the release of angiotensin I which is rapidly hydrolysed to angiotensin II. The latter in addition to its pressor action stimulates aldosterone secretion which then acts on the distal tubules to produce sodium retention.

3. True
The positive sodium balance induced by adrenal cortical aldosterone secretion increases the volume of extracellular water and in addition enhances the pressor activity of angiotensin.

4. True
Renin, by way of angiotensin, has a pressor effect which is mediated mainly by peripheral vasoconstriction.

5. False
This system has no direct effect on nitrogen balance.

20.4 The blood urea is elevated in the following conditions:
1. severe dehydration
2. pregnancy
3. tubular necrosis
4. diabetes insipidus
5. cortical necrosis

1. True
Severe dehydration eventually leads to a fall in the effective blood volume which is followed by hypotension and a diminution in the renal perfusion. At first a physiological diminution in the urine output occurs which can be corrected if the underlying dehydration is rapidly and effectively dealt with. If, however, the condition is not corrected tubular or cortical necrosis follows.

2. False
In pregnancy a low blood urea is commonplace because of the relative increase in blood volume.

3. True
Tubular necrosis is followed by severe oliguria and the retention of urea. Rarely the volume of urine may be as great or greater than normal but urea retention still occurs. This condition is known as non-oliguric renal failure and is particularly seen following severe burns.

4. False
Diabetes insipidus, caused by damage to the hypothalamus or the posterior portion of the hypophysis, is normally not associated with changes in the blood urea.

5. True
Cortical necrosis is followed by an immediate rise in blood urea and anuria. The condition is irreversible and requires intermittent dialysis or renal transplantation to maintain life.

20.5 Combined water and electrolyte depletion causes:
1. a high concentration of sodium in the urine
2. a high urine specific gravity
3. pre-renal uraemia
4. a fall in the central venous pressure
5. a high blood urea nitrogen to creatinine ratio

1. False
A combined water and electrolyte depletion results in an augmented secretion of aldosterone which causes an increase in the tubular reabsorption of sodium and hence a low urinary sodium concentration.

2. True
The conservation of water by the kidney results in the excretion of a hypertonic urine. The specific gravity rises above 1020 and the osmolality exceeds 500 mOsm/l.

3. True
The diminishing blood volume results in a gradual decline in renal perfusion and hence a diminished excretion of urea. The retention of urea eventually leads to pre-renal uraemia.

4. True
The decrease in blood volume eventually leads to a decline in the

central venous pressure following the exhaustion of the compensatory mechanisms.

5. False

The pre-renal uraemia associated with water and electrolyte depletion causes a disproportionate rise in the blood urea nitrogen as compared to the rising concentration of creatinine. The normal ratio between these substances is 10:1 but in severe depletion may rise to levels as high as 20 or 25:1.

20.6 Pure water depletion in the surgical patient follows:

1. persistent vomiting
2. dysphagia
3. severe diarrhoea
4. persistent fever
5. the development of diabetes insipidus

1. False

Persistent vomiting results in a combined water and electrolyte depletion because of the electrolytes present in the gastrointestinal juices. Gastric juice, for example, contains between 70 and 140 mEq/l (mmol/l) of sodium and between 5 and 40 mEq/l (mmol/l) of potassium.

2. True

Dysphagia caused by benign or malignant strictures of the oesophagus results, if sufficiently severe, in the regurgitation of all water taken by mouth in addition to the loss of saliva. The result is a pure water depletion because fluid rather than electrolytes is lost.

3. False

Severe diarrhoea gives rise to a combined depletion in which the loss of potassium is of great importance because diarrhoeal stools contain between 10 and 40 mEq/l (10 to 40 mmol/l) of this cation. The loss of approximately 10% of the total body potassium causes the serum potassium to fall from 4 mEq/l (mmol/l) to 3 mEq/l (mmol/l) at a normal pH.

4. True

Fever is associated with increased sweating. This is the major mechanism of heat loss but is only effective if the sweat evaporates on the skin surface, thus extracting the latent heat of vaporisation. Excessive sweating causes a pure water depletion but if the water alone is replaced salt deficiency follows.

5. True

Diabetes insipidus follows a reduction, from whatever cause, of circulating vasopressin. A vasopressin deficiency results in the excretion of large volumes of dilute urine due to an alteration in the response of the tubular cells to the movement of water. Between 5 and 10 litres/day of urine may be excreted daily leading rapidly, unless corrected, by a corresponding increase in water intake, to water depletion.

20.7 The metabolic effects following a severe injury include:
1. respiratory alkalosis
2. accelerated gluconeogenesis
3. mobilisation of fat stores
4. decreased aldosterone secretion
5. protein anabolism

1. True
Respiratory alkalosis may follow the hyperventilation induced by pain and blood loss.

2. True
Afferent stimuli reaching the central nervous system through large neurons causes the hypothalamus to secrete corticotrophin releasing factor (CRF). The resulting stimulation of the anterior pituitary releases adrenotrophic hormone (ACTH). This, in turn, stimulates the excessive secretion of glucocorticoids by the adrenal cortex which accelerates gluconeogenesis and increases the deposition of liver glycogen.

3. True
The mobilisation of fat stores from adipose tissue elevates the serum levels of free fatty acids. The net effect is to increase the plasma concentration of carbohydrate and lipid intermediates producing the 'diabetes of injury'.

4. False
Aldosterone secretion may be increased almost thirty-fold following severe trauma. This enhances the renal tubular absorption of sodium thus helping to maintain the extracellular fluid volume. In addition the excretion of hydrogen ion and potassium are increased thus delaying the onset of a metabolic acidosis and hyperkalaemia.

5. False
Trauma from whatever cause induces protein catabolism. Normally an individual receiving no protein in the diet excretes nitrogen at an accelerated rate of 10 to 12 g/day for about 14 days after which a gradual decline occurs. In contrast, following major trauma and in the same dietary conditions the excretion of nitrogen may reach 20 g/day and if in addition there is superadded sepsis the nitrogen excretion may reach 30 g/day. This is equivalent to the loss of 180 g of protein daily or 1 kg (wet weight) of body tissue.

20.8 Hyperkalaemia commonly occurs:
1. following severe burns
2. in Conn's syndrome
3. following glomerular necrosis

4. in the Zollinger–Ellison syndrome
5. in the carcinoid syndrome

1. True
Hyperkalaemia occurs in severe burns due to the following factors:
 (a) Liberation of potassium from the haemolysis of the
   erythrocytes destroyed or damaged in the burnt area
 (b) Associated tissue catabolism
 (c) Retention of potassium due to renal failure

2. False
This uncommon syndrome, which is usually caused by aldosterone secreting tumours of the adrenal cortex, is associated with the retention of sodium and the excessive excretion of potassium leading to hypokalaemia.

3. True
Glomerular necrosis, however caused, results in irreversible renal failure and the retention of potassium.

4. False
The Zollinger–Ellison syndrome caused by gastrin secreting tumours of the islet cells of the pancreas may be associated with severe diarrhoea. Should this occur water and electrolyte depletion follows and hyperkalaemia would only occur if secondary renal failure developed.

5. False
The carcinoid syndrome may be associated with diarrhoea but this is normally episodic and rarely sufficiently severe to produce electrolyte depletion.

20.9 Hypocalcaemia occurs:
 1. following surgical damage or removal of the parathyroid glands
 2. following fractures of the long bones
 3. during attacks of acute pancreatitis
 4. following head injury
 5. in association with hypomagnesaemia

1. True
Hypocalcaemia follows damage to the parathyroid glands during the operation of thyroidectomy. Some surgeons argue that the cause is removal of the glands, others that it is due to damage to their arterial supply leading to infarction. Whatever the precise cause the end result is a diminished supply of parathyroid hormone and tetany follows.

2. False
Simple fractures of the long bones do not affect the serum calcium.

3. True
Severe pancreatitis is associated with the liberation of the enzyme, lipase. This specifically hydrolyses fat, especially within the

abdomen, the liberated soaps combine with calcium causing acute hypocalcaemia. If this does occur in pancreatitis it is regarded as a bad prognostic sign.

4. False
Although severe trauma may be associated with hypocalcaemia head injury alone does not produce this metabolic disturbance.

5. True
Hypomagnesaemia is frequently associated with hypocalcaemia. This is due to the fact that both electrolyte disturbances may share a common aetiology, i.e. malabsorption from whatever cause.

20.10 Severe pyloric stenosis is accompanied by the following biochemical changes:
1. a fall in the effective blood volume
2. a fall in the concentration of plasma sodium
3. a rise in pCO_2
4. hypotonic urine
5. hyperkalaemia

1. True
The continuous loss of water accompanied by sodium and chloride reduces the volume of all fluid spaces including the blood volume. The net result on the kidney is renal vasoconstriction and a reduced glomerular filtration rate and as a result the blood urea is elevated.

2. False
Although there is an overall sodium deficiency due to vomiting the vomitus contains relatively more water than sodium so that the concentration of plasma sodium sometimes rises. If, however, the patient is allowed to drink, the selective partial replacement of water to the exclusion of sodium lowers the plasma concentration of sodium below normal.

3. True
The loss of hydrogen ions raises the plasma pH, slows respiration and raises the pCO_2.

4. False
The normal change in the urine is oliguria associated with a hypertonic urine. If renal ischaemia is severe tubular necrosis follows.

5. False
The continuous vomiting leads to a low plasma potassium and to compensate for this a potassium shift occurs from the intracellular space to the plasma and extracellular space, together with a reverse shift of hydrogen and sodium ions from the extracellular space into the cells.

SECTION 21. BLOOD TRANSFUSION

21.1 Blood which is to be used for transfusion:
1. should be stored at –4°C
2. may need to be irradiated (1000 r)
3. needs to be tested for complement content
4. may be used after storage for platelet replacement
5. should be stored in an acid anticoagulant

1. False
Blood transfusion should be stored at +4°C. If frozen the erythrocytes will be lysed releasing haemoglobin into the plasma. The introduction of lysed blood into a recipient can give rise to an immediate transfusion reaction accompanied by haemoglobinaemia, haemoglobinuria and possibly oliguria followed by acute renal failure.

2. True
Fresh blood transfused to an immunodeficient patient should be irradiated to prevent a graft versus host reaction.

3. False
Stored blood does not contain very much active complement and is not normally checked for circulating immune complexes.

4. False
If platelet replacement is required fresh blood must be used as platelets decay rapidly. Platelet transfusions are required in cases of bone marrow aplasia and acute leukaemia. If, however, platelet autoantibodies have developed or if increased destruction of platelets is occurring in the spleen, platelet transfusion will be ineffective.

5. True
The standard anticoagulant used for donor blood is acid citrate dextrose. This is a mixture of citric acid, trisodium citrate and dextrose, acidification increasing the preserving power of the solution.

21.2 The following tests should be performed on donor blood before it is used for transfusion:
1. HBsAg
2. Van den Bergh
3. Wassermann test or the VDRL flocculation test
4. acid phosphatase
5. malaria smear

1. True
The presence of HBsAg (Australia antigen) in donor blood means that there is a high risk of transferring hepatitis B infection to the recipient. This antigen may be identified by a variety of methods including gel precipitation and counterimmuno-electrophoresis.

2. False
The Van den Bergh diazo test for bilirubin is not routinely performed on donor blood prior to transfusion.

3. True
In the presence of a positive Wassermann or VDRL flocculation reaction there is a risk of the transfused blood transferring syphilis. Thus Wassermann or VDRL positive blood should not be used for transfusion.

4. False
The acid phosphatase in serum is raised in prostatic cancer with osteoplastic secondary deposits in bone.

5. True
In tropical countries in which malaria is endemic there is always a risk of transfusing blood containing malaria parasites; a smear should, therefore, be examined to exclude this disease in donor blood.

21.3   The following refer to blood group antigens:
1. Lewis
2. Von Willebrand
3. Duffy
4. Turner
5. Kidd

1. True
Lewis antigens Le^a and Le^b associated with the red cells are also found in the saliva and plasma. The system is controlled by the genes Le and le. There is a connection between the Lewis system and the ability to secrete blood group substances. Lewis antibodies are not associated with haemolytic disease of the newborn since they belong to the IgM group and, therefore, cannot cross the placenta.

2. False
Von Willebrand's disease is a hereditary clotting disorder similar to haemophilia. The deficiency is in clotting Factor VIII but, in addition, an increased bleeding time occurs due to capillary fragility. Clinically, the condition presents with mucosal bleeding as well as repeated attacks of haemarthrosis.

3. True
The Duffy system (Fy^a positive and Fy^a negative) give rise to IgG antibodies that can pass across the placenta and give rise to haemolytic disease of the newborn. Anti-Fy^a antibodies are best detected by a Coombs test.

4. False
Turner's syndrome is due to the absence of the Y chromosome and a single X chromosome. It is associated with ovarian dysgenesis, a lack of sexual development and a webbed neck.

5. True

The Kidd system (Jk^a positive and Jk^a negative) is similar to the Duffy and Kell blood group systems. These antigens can also result in IgG antibodies causing severe haemolytic disease of the newborn.

21.4 An immediate reaction to a blood transfusion may be caused by the following:
1. hypercalcaemia
2. air embolus
3. bacterial endotoxins
4. anaphylaxis
5. hypokalaemia

1. False

A transfusion of blood does not give rise to hypercalcaemia. However, the transfusion of large volumes of stored blood may give rise to hypocalcaemia due to the action of the citrate which is used as an anticoagulant. This effect can be reversed by the administration of calcium gluconate.

2. True

Air embolus is a recognised risk of any transfusion administered by a donor set with interchangeable parts. Much of this risk has been removed by the use of plastic packs.

3. True

Fever was a common complication of blood transfusion in the past. It arose either because the blood had been contaminated by bacterial endotoxins or because residual pyrogens had been absorbed onto the donor apparatus. Many of these latter reactions have been eliminated by the use of plastic disposable donor sets.

4. True

Anaphylactic reaction following transfusion gives rise to urticaria. The responsible antigens are probably derived from food ingested immediately prior to taking the blood, examples being bovine milk and egg proteins.

5. False

Massive transfusions lead to hyperkalaemia, this can cause heart failure and possibly sudden death.

21.5 The physical results of Rhesus incompatibility include the following:
1. hydrops fetalis
2. Hutchinson's teeth
3. icterus neonatorum
4. hepato-lenticular degeneration
5. kernicterus

1. True

Severe Rhesus incompatibility results in hydrops fetalis, a cause of intrauterine death due to the development of marked anaemia and congestive heart failure, the latter causing severe oedema, hence the name.

2. False

Hutchinson's teeth have no connection with Rhesus incompatibility, they are one of the many stigmata of congenital syphilis.

3. True

Extreme incompatibility causes such a severe degree of intravascular haemolysis that the affected baby is deeply jaundiced at birth.

4. False

Hepato-lenticular degeneration, Wilson's disease, has no connection with Rhesus incompatibility. It is a familial disease of children caused by an excess of free copper in the circulation due to the low levels of the copper binding caeruloplasmin in the circulation. Copper is deposited in the brain particularly in the putamen and caudate nucleus and also in the liver and kidneys.

5. True

The severe haemolysis which may occur in Rhesus incompatibility results in jaundice causing the condition known as kernicterus in which staining of the hippocampus and basal nuclei with bile occurs This leads to localized brain damage with necrosis of the affected neurons which is later followed by gliosis. If not fatal the child is likely to suffer from choreoathetosis, spasticity and mental deficiency.

21.6 Haemolytic disease of the newborn:
1. may be caused by *Treponema pallidum*
2. may be due to anti-c
3. may occur in the first pregnancy
4. frequently is not found until the second pregnancy
5. can be treated with anti-D antibodies

1. False

Treponema pallidum plays no part in haemolytic disease of the newborn which is chiefly caused by Rhesus incompatibility and rarely to ABO incompatibility.

2. True

Rhesus incompatibility is usually due to anti-D but rarely it can be due to either anti-c or anti-E.

3. True

HDN can occur in the first pregnancy but only if the mother has previously received an Rh incompatible transfusion.

4. True

The first pregnancy is usually uneventful, the Rh- mother being delivered of a normal Rh+ fetus without any apparent difficulty.

However, the Rh- mother is sensitised to the Rh+ red cells by fetal cells leaking across the placenta into the maternal circulation, which are then recognised by the maternal immune system leading to the development of IgG immunoglobulins postpartum which cross the placenta in subsequent pregnancies. Thus the second and subsequent fetuses are at increasing risk of developing HDNB.

5. True

The idea that HDNB could be prevented by the administration of anti RhD antibodies arose from the observation that there is a lower incidence of the condition if the father is of different ABO group to the mother. This led to the idea that Rh+ fetal red cells would be rapidly destroyed in an Rh- mother by preformed antibodies if the mother and child were ABO incompatible. Destroyed, they would not be available to sensitise the maternal immune system to RhD antigen. This forms the basis for Rh prophylaxis in which anti-RhD antibodies are given to an Rh- mother immediately after delivery.

21.7 The Coombs test is used for detecting:
1. rheumatoid factor
2. antinuclear factor
3. haemolytic autoantibodies
4. cold agglutinins
5. Rhesus antibodies

1. False

The Coombs test uses an antihuman globulin antibody to detect specific immunoglobulins or complement attached to, or capable of attaching to, the surface of human erythrocytes. The rheumatoid factor is, however, an antibody directed towards the Gm groups on the Fc fragment of immunoglobulins. It is detected either by using sensitised sheep erythrocytes (Rose–Waaler test) or latex particles onto which human IgG has been absorbed.

2. False

The antinuclear factor is an autoantibody chiefly present in the serum of patients suffering from systemic lupus erythematosus. It is detected either by a latex test in which the antigen is absorbed onto latex particles or by immunofluorescent techniques.

3. True

The direct Coombs test detects antibodies that have already reacted with antigen on the red cell surface. The indirect Coombs test is used to detect antibodies to red cell antigens present in serum which are first reacted with specific red cells before the application of antihuman globulin reagent. The test produces red cell agglutination. The Coombs test differentiates the immune haemolytic anaemias from all other forms of haemolytic anaemia by detecting anti-red cell antibodies.

4. True
The Coombs test will detect agglutinins that have reacted with the surface of the erythrocyte even if the reaction occurs at 37°C.

5. True
The presence of IgG (incomplete) Rhesus antibodies in the serum can be detected by the use of an indirect Coombs test.

21.8 The following antibodies may pass across the placenta:
1. anti A isohaemagglutinin
2. immune antiblood group A
3. anti D (Rhesus)
4. diphtheria antitoxin
5. rheumatoid factor

1. False
The anti ABO blood group antibodies present in normal plasma are IgM antibodies (MW 900 000) too large to pass across the placenta.

2. True
The immune anti ABO blood group antibodies which may develop after a transfusion of incompatible blood are sometimes of IgG type and may, therefore, pass across the placenta to cause haemolytic disease of the newborn.

3. True
Anti D (Rhesus) antibodies formed following Rhesus positive pregnancies in Rhesus negative mothers or an incompatible transfusion in a Rhesus negative mother are usually of IgG type and, therefore, pass across the placenta.

4. True
Diphtheria antitoxin is an IgG antibody which, therefore, passes across the placenta.

5. False
The rheumatoid factor is an IgM anti IgG autoantibody developing in individuals suffering from rheumatoid arthritis and does not pass across the placenta.

SECTION 22. IONISING IRRADIATION AND CYTOTOXIC AGENTS

22.1 Ionising radiation:
1. increases DNA synthesis
2. increases H_2O_2 in the tissues
3. breaks disulphide bonds
4. causes atrophy of the seminiferous tubules of the testis
5. causes pathological fractures

1. False

The direct effect of irradiation is to produce single or double stranded chromosomal breaks leading to the formation of cross linkages which impair the ability of DNA to act as a template.

2. True

This is called the indirect effect of irradiation. Oxidising compounds such as H_2O_2 are formed. This gives rise to the oxidation of -SH groups to -S-S- groups.

3. False

Disulphide bonds are formed rather than broken following irradiation. This causes the inactivation of enzymes which contain -SH groups as part of their biochemically active sites.

4. True

The first effect of irradiation on the testes is the destruction of the spermatogonia. A later effect is atrophy of the seminiferous tubules.

5. True

In the fetus and the child prior to fusion of the epiphyses, bone and cartilage are radiosensitive with the result that skeletal distortion may occur. In the adult, the effects of irradiation are indirect and are caused by changes in the blood vessels followed by their occlusion leading to bone necrosis.

22.2   The effect(s) of ionising irradiation:
1. are increased by sulphydryl reagents
2. are increased by increased oxygen tension
3. is mainly upon mitochondria
4. is to cause diarrhoea
5. is to cause a deficiency of clotting factors

1. False

See answer to question 2.

2. True

An increase in the oxygen tension in the environment of a malignant tumour increases the tumoricidal effects of irradiation. Much of this effect is believed to be caused by the oxidation of the -SH groups of enzymes to -S-S- groups, thus inactivating enzyme activity. In animal tumour systems sulphydryl containing compounds such as cysteine, cyteamine and AET afford some protection from the effects of irradiation. Unfortunately this effect has had no beneficial effect on the outcome of human cancer treatment.

3. False

There is no doubt that irradiation has an effect on the mitochondrial enzymes but its major effect is to inhibit DNA synthesis and mitosis, thus the main effect of ionising irradiation on any cell is at a nuclear level.

4. True
Apart from the oesophagus and rectum, the mid portion of the gastrointestinal tract is very radiosensitive, particularly the crypt cells of the small intestine with their high cell turnover rate. A whole body dose between 600–100 rem causes nausea, vomiting and diarrhoea.

5. False
Ionising irradiation may be followed by severe bleeding but if this occurs it is due to a platelet deficiency caused by a direct radiation effect on the megakaryocytes of the bone marrow. Following a whole body dose of between 400–600 rem platelet depression associated with severe bleeding occurs within 3–5 weeks.

22.3 Ionising radiation:
  1. does not affect the eyes
  2. affects renal function
  3. does not affect the lungs
  4. affects the brain
  5. does not affect the skin

1. False
Large doses of irradiation, particularly by neutrons, cause cataracts.

2. True
Excessive exposure of the kidneys to ionising irradiation causes first acute tubule injury followed by a progressive glomerular fibrosis which leads to malignant hypertension and a progressive diminution of renal function.

3. False
Ionising irradiation does affect lungs causing pulmonary fibrosis and a decline in respiratory function. This was a relatively common complication following the treatment of carcinoma of the breast prior to the use of high energy irradiation and tangential fields.

4. True
Very high doses in excess of 5000 r may be associated with cerebral syndrome in which hyperthermia followed by a state of shock occurs.

5. False
Ionising irradiation gives rise to an inflammatory response which is later followed by atrophy of the skin and hypopigmentation and subsequently the development of squamous carcinomata, and/or rodent ulcers.

22.4 The following are immunosuppressive drugs:
  1. azathioprine
  2. indomethacin
  3. oxyprenolol
  4. cyclophosphamide
  5. chlorpropamide

1. True
Azathioprine, a guanine analogue based on 6-mercaptopurine, is a widely used immunosuppressive drug in clinical practice. It is part of the standard drug regime used to prevent graft rejection in renal transplantation patients and it is also occasionally used in the treatment of autoimmune diseases such as systemic lupus erythematosus.

2. False
Indomethacin is an anti-inflammatory drug without any direct immunosuppressive action. It is chiefly used in the treatment of rheumatoid arthritis. Indomethacin inhibits the formation of prostaglandins from the substrate arachidonic acid.

3. False
Oxyprenolol and propanolol are β adrenergic receptor blockers and are used in the treatment of cardiac arrhythmias and hypertension.

4. True
Cyclophosphamide is an alkylating agent derived from nitrogen mustard. As a cytotoxic drug it is chiefly used in the treatment of neoplastic disease but it is cytotoxic to all rapidly dividing cells and, therefore, to the lymphocytes concerned in the immune response, although it is not particularly effective in preventing graft rejection.

5. False
Chlorpropamide is an oral antidiabetic agent. It reduces the blood sugar by increasing the cellular uptake of glucose and decreasing the intestinal absorption of sugars.

22.5 The following compounds may be used as anti-cancer agents:
1. azathioprine
2. methotrexate
3. actinomycin D
4. chlorambucil
5. cyclosporin A

1. False
Azathioprine (Imuran) is an immunosuppressive agent which is commonly used to suppress transplant rejection and occasionally for the treatment of autoimmune immune complex diseases, such as systemic lupus erythematosus. It is not an anticancer agent.

2. True
Methotrexate is a folic acid inhibitor used in the treatment of leukaemia. It has also been used as an immunosuppressive agent and also to suppress the epidermal proliferation which occurs in psoriasis.

3. True
The actinomycins are antibiotics which suppress proliferating tissue in man. Actinomycin D selectively complexes with DNA and thus

inhibits RNA and protein synthesis. This antibiotic is particularly effective in the treatment of childhood renal tumours. Actinomycin C which contains some actinomycin D has been used in combination with azathioprine to prevent the rejection of renal transplants.

4. True
Aminophenylbutyric acid mustard (chlorambucil) is an alkylating agent which has been used to suppress cellular and particularly neoplastic proliferation.

5. False
Cyclosporin A is a fungal metabolite which acts as an immunosuppressive agent by its actions on the T lymphocytes. It has been used to treat renal allograft recipients and to prevent graft versus host disease after bone marrow transplantation.

22.6 The following compounds are alkylating agents:
1. azathioprine
2. methotrexate
3. cyclophosphamide
4. phenylalanine mustard
5. tetracycline

1. False
Azathioprine (Imuran) is the carrier form of 6-mercaptopurine which is incorporated into DNA instead of guanine as a fraudulent base.

2. False
Methotrexate is a folic acid inhibitor blocking DNA synthesis.

3. True
Cyclophosphamide is not strictly an alkylating agent but it is broken down by the liver in vivo to liberate nitrogen mustard which is an alkylating agent.

4. True
L phenyl alanine mustard (Melphalan) is an alkylating agent. Great hopes were once entertained that this drug would be successful in the cure of malignant melanoma because it was considered that the phenyl alanine would be incorporated into the melanoma cells as a precursor of melanin. These high hopes were soon dashed.

5. False
Tetracycline is a broad spectrum antibiotic prepared from chlortetracycline, its action is that of a bacteriostatic agent.

22.7 The following immunosuppressive agents are purine or pyrimidine analogues:
1. cyclosporine
2. azathioprine
3. methotrexate

4. actinomycin C
5. prednisone

1. False
As stated in 25.5.5 cyclosporine is a fungal metabolite unrelated to the alkylating agents. Cyclosporine suppresses T cell-mediated immunity by inhibiting activation of cytokine genes, in particular IL-2. It has had a major impact on organ transplantation. Unfortunately, prolonged immunosuppression gives rise to a greater than normal incidence of malignancy, most frequently, immunoblastic B-cell lymphomas. It also causes renal damage.

2. True
Azathioprine, which is commonly used following renal transplantation, is a derivative of 6-mercaptopurine which is an analogue of the purine base guanine, disturbing the DNA sequence which following this cannot be transcribed, thus effectively blocking protein synthesis. Apart from the possibility of malignancy following long term suppression, azathioprine may produce interstitial pneumonitis.

3. False
Methotrexate is a folic acid analogue blocking the action of the enzyme folic reductase. As a result, dihydrofolinic acid cannot be reduced to tetrahydrofolinic acid. This is a necessary step for the conversion of uracil desoxyriboside to thymidine, the latter being an essential constituent of DNA.

4. False
Actinomycin C is an antibiotic derived from cultures of *Streptomyces antibioticus*. It selectively competes with DNA inhibiting RNA and protein synthesis. This agent was in the past used to supplement azathioprine in renal transplantation and one of its components actinomycin D is still used for the treatment of renal tumours of childhood.

5. False
Prednisone is a glucocorticoid. The mechanism by which glucocorticoids act as immunosuppressive agents in man is poorly understood. However, they have a strong anti-inflammatory component.

22.8 Chlorambucil, a potent cytotoxic agent, causes:
   1. bone marrow depression
   2. indirect interference with mitosis
   3. inhibition of purine synthesis
   4. binding of DNA strands
   5. inhibition of protein synthesis

1. True
Bone marrow depression is common to all cytotoxic agents since the doubling time of the stem cells in the bone marrow is only 15–20

hours, whereas in a tumour system the doubling time may be as long as 500 days. The first noticeable toxic effect is on the white cells, the life span of which is only 4–5 days. When the absolute granulocyte count falls below 10 g/L the patient is at risk of infection especially with opportunistic or endogenous organisms.

2. True
By binding the DNA strands together chlorambucil indirectly interferes with mitosis, see **4**. This action should be compared to the mode of action of the vinca alkaloids which arrest cell division at the metaphase probably by interfering with spindle formation so that the chromatids cannot be properly paired.

3. False
The chief inhibitors of purine synthesis are the nitrosoureas which block the enzymes responsible for purine synthesis and the incorporation of purine into DNA.

4. True
Chlorambucil is an alkylating agent and its cytotoxicity is effected by the development of cross linkages or bridges between opposite guanine bases. This binds the DNA strands together and prevents them from separating at the time of division.

5. True
Inhibition of protein synthesis is an essential feature of the action of all alkylating cytotoxic agents.

22.9   DNA synthesis is inhibited by:
1. prednisone
2. methane sulphonic acid
3. methotrexate
4. azathioprine
5. chloramphenicol

1. False
Glucocorticoids do not directly affect DNA synthesis. They are neither antimitotic agents nor inhibitors of protein synthesis.

2. True
Methane sulphonic acid (Busulphan), is an alkylating agent used in cancer chemotherapy. This agent is believed to form alkyl bridges across the DNA double helix thus inhibiting normal DNA replication.

3. True
Methotrexate is an inhibitor of folic acid which binds the enzyme, folic reductase, thus preventing the reduction of dihydrofolinic acid to tetrahydrofolinic acid. The latter acts as a coenzyme for the conversion of uracil desoxyriboside into thymidine, which is necessary for DNA synthesis.

4. True
Azathioprine (Imuran) is a carrier form of 6-mercaptopurine. It is

incorporated into the DNA molecule as a 'fraudulent' base in place of guanine thus preventing the normal synthesis of DNA.

5. False
Chloramphenicol is a broad spectrum antibiotic which was originally obtained from *Streptomyces venezuelae* but is now artificially synthesized. It prevents protein synthesis by mammalian cells by blocking the formation of peptide chains from amino acids on the ribosomes. In addition it may also block the synthesis of messenger RNA in proliferating cells.

SECTION 23. TRANSPLANTATION AND HIV

23.1 The chief effector cells involved in the rejection of a renal allograft are:
   1. CD4+ T cells
   2. CD8+ T cells
   3. passenger leucocytes
   4. platelets
   5. B lymphocytes

1. True
The importance of these cells is shown by the finding that 'nude' mice and rats which have a congenital lack of CD4+ T cells require no immunosuppression.

2. True
These cells cause lysis of the renal parenchymal cells.

3. True
Passenger leucocytes (dendritic cells) act in the initial phase of sensitisation without which rejection would not be initiated. They are present in the graft and carry high concentrations of donor MHC molecules recognised by the recipient's CD4+ cells.

4. False
Platelets play no part in the rejection process.

5. False
B cells play no part in the effector phase of rejection.

23.2 The virus associated with HIV is:
   1. an obligate intracellular virus
   2. a commoner infection in haemophiliacs than in normal individuals
   3. transmitted from mother to infant
   4. related to the visna virus which infects sheep
   5. a single genetic form

1. True
This is the significant difference between bacterial and viral infections. All viruses infecting man are obligate intracellular organisms multiplying within the living cell.

2. False
Normally HIV infection is not more common in haemophiliacs than in normal individuals, but outbreaks have occurred in this group of people due to them receiving contaminated blood products.

3. True
Mother to infant infection can be transmitted either via the placental blood, during delivery or by ingestion of infected breast milk.

4. True
HIV is a retrovirus belonging to the lentovirus family; included within this group is the visna virus of sheep.

5. False
There are two genetically different but related forms of HIV, HIV1 and HIV2. HIV1 is common in Central Africa, whereas HIV2 is common in West Africa.

23.3 Acute graft versus host disease following bone marrow transplantation is followed by damage to:
1. the skin
2. the gut
3. the brain
4. the liver
5. the endocrine glands

1. True
AGVHD is characterized by dermatitis. The skin eruption takes the form of pruritic macular areas on the palms and soles with moniliform lesions of the extremities, trunk and face.

2. True
In the gastrointestinal tract, crypt cell necrosis with marked lymphocytic infiltration occurs. The diagnosis can be made by rectal biopsy.

3. False
The brain is never involved.

4. True
Damage to the liver occurs between 10–50 days after the transplantation. It is dominated by a direct attack of the donor lymphocytes on the hepatocytes and the bile duct epithelium, producing a hepoatitic picture.

5. False
The endocrine glands do not appear to be damaged.

23.4 AIDS encephalopathy is:
1. an infrequent feature of the disease
2. mainly affects the grey matter
3. associated with rarefaction and vacuolation
4. associated with mental retardation in children
5. caused by CD4+ T-cell deficiency

1. False
About 40% of AIDS patients have neurological symptoms and 80% have pathological changes in the CNS at autopsy, changes which are due to the direct or indirect effects of the virus, opportunistic infection and primary CNS lymphoma.

2. False
The white matter and basal ganglia are chiefly affected.

3. True
Rarefaction and vacuolation are associated with the destruction of myelin sheaths and disruption of some axons. Infiltration with macrophages and multinucleate cells may be found.

4. True
Almost half of the infants and children infected with HIV develop an encephalopathy which leads to mental retardation and motor dysfunction.

5. False
These changes are thought to be the direct result of viral infection and unrelated to a defect in cell-mediated immunity.

23.5 Immunosuppression can be achieved by:
1. cyclosporine
2. rapamycin
3. monoclonal antibodies
4. poor renal function
5. blood transfusion prior to surgery

1. True
The introduction of cyclosporine produced a great advance in transplant surgery. Cyclosporine is a fungal macrolide which affects the production of lymphokines by the T cells.

2. True
Rapamycin is another fungal derivative which causes immunosuppression by interfering with the action of IL-2.

3. True
Various monoclonal antibodies have been produced which act in different ways e.g. Anti CD3 acts on mature T cells, Anti CD4 acts on T helper cells and Anti CD25 acts on activated T cells.

4. True
As renal function fails, so a non-specific atrophy of all lymphoid tissue occurs due to the development of uraemia.

5. True
It has been shown that prior transfusion increases the percentage of graft survival. How this is achieved is possibly by the selective activation of Th cells or by the activation of T cells.

23.6 Kaposi sarcoma is:
1. not as common as non-Hodgkin's lymphoma in patients suffering from AIDS
2. different in the sporadic form from that occurring in AIDS
3. histologically identical in both the sporadic and AIDS-related forms
4. not associated with transplantation
5. related to haemangiosarcoma

1. False
Non-Hodgkin's lymphoma is less common in the end stage of AIDS than is Kaposi sarcoma. Approximately 3% of AIDS patients develop lymphoma whereas one third develop a Kaposi sarcoma.

2. True
Sporadic Kaposi sarcoma occurs especially in Ashkenazi Jews, forming red nodules principally on the lower extremities, whereas AIDS-related Kaposi sarcoma has no such specific site, disseminating widely.

3. True
The two types, sporadic and AIDS-related, cannot be distinguished histologically.

4. False
High doses of immune suppressive drugs in transplant patients may be followed by the development of Kaposi sarcoma.

5. False
Haemangiosarcoma are rare tumours which may be associated with exposure to arsenical pesticides and polyvinyl chloride which is widely used in the plastic industry.

23.7 The following grafts are rejected:
1. autografts
2. isografts
3. allografts
4. xenografts
5. corneal grafts

1. False
Transplantation of an individual's own tissue to another site, e.g. the

covering of a full thickness burn with skin from an unburnt area, is not rejected.

2. False
Transplantation of tissues between genetically identical members of the same species, e.g. kidney transplants between monozygotic twins or skin grafts between mice of the same inbred strain, are not rejected.

3. True
Transplantation between genetically non-identical members of the same species, e.g. a cadaveric renal transplant or a skin graft between mice of different inbred strains are rejected.

4. True
Transplantation of tissues between members of different species are rejected.

5. False
The cornea is in an immunologically privileged site.

23.8 HIV infection is associated with:+
1. a reduction in the number of B cells
2. hypergammaglobulinaemia
3. increased tuberculin skin test reactivity
4. cytokine abnormalities
5. autoimmunity

1. False
There is profound depletion of CD4+ T lymphocytes. B-lymphocyte function may only be affected in that it may depend on T helper cell function.

2. True
There is a polyclonal hypergammaglobulinaemia resulting from non-specific stimulation of B cells.

3. False
Delayed hypersensitivity is reduced or absent due to depletion of T cells.

4. True
There is reduced production of cytokines produced by CD4+ T cells, such as IL-2 and gamma-interferon.

5. False
There is no evidence that HIV infection predisposes to autoimmunity.

23.9 Chronic renal allograft rejection is a process:
1. affecting about 10–30% of long-surviving grafts
2. characterized by proliferative stenosis of the arteries
3. in which cellular infiltrates and fibrinoid necrosis occurs

4. can be reversed by medical treatment
5. requires graft replacement

1. True
Approximately 10–30% of long-surviving grafts are finally rejected.

2. True
Whereas acute rejection is characterized by cellular infiltration and fibrinoid necrosis, chronic rejection is characterized by proliferative stenosing lesions of arteries.

3. False
Cellular infiltration does occur, but it is abnormal typically arterial obliteration which causes renal failure in chronic rejection.

4. False
The process once begun cannot be reversed.

5. True
Because medical treatment cannot affect the gradual stenosis of the renal arteries, the only treatment available is to remove the graft and possibly regraft later.

23.10 Hyperacute rejection is:
1. a condition associated with a T-cell mediated reaction
2. a condition recognised at operation
3. associated with the Schwartzmann reaction
4. a condition mediated by preformed antibodies
5. a condition seen in multiparous women

1. False
Hyperacute rejection occurs in the presence of preformed antidonor antibodies in the circulation of the recipient.

2. True
In hyperacute rejection, the phenomenon occurs so rapidly that it is almost instantly recognised. In renal transplantation following the restitution of the vascular supply, the kidney instead of becoming pink and excreting urine becomes cyanosed, mottled and may excrete only a few drops of bloody urine.

3. False
The histological changes resemble those of the Arthus reaction, in which immunofluorescent studies show that after the initial deposition of antigen (in the case of transplantation the donor organ), deposition of antibody (already preformed) and complement occurs in the arterioles and peritubular capillaries, followed by an intravascular clumping of platelets.

4. True
The reaction is mediated by antibodies rather than T cells.

5. True

Preformed donor antibodies may be present in a patient who has already received and rejected a homograft and they may also be present in multiparous women who develop anti-HLA antibodies against paternal antigens shed from the fetus; these may cause a hyperacute rejection to grafts taken from their husbands or children.

23.11 Which of the following statements regarding HIV infection is true:

1. infection with HIV is followed by a short incubation period and by a rapidly progressive illness ending in a fatal outcome
2. it is associated with the formation of giant cells
3. the virus expresses specific trophism for the haemopoetic and nervous systems
4. the risk of infection by blood transfusion has been completely eliminated
5. the virus is surrounded by a lipid membrane

1. False

Characteristically all retroviral infections are followed by a long incubation period and a slowly progressive fatal outcome.

2. True

The fusion of infected and uninfected cells leads to the formation of giant cells which usually die within a few hours.

3. True

The retroviruses exhibit marked trophism for the haemopoetic and the nervous systems.

4. False

Even with present day screening a very slight risk of infection remains, since a recently infected individual may be antibody negative at the time of giving blood.

5. True

The virion is spherical and contains an electron dense core surrounded by a lipid envelope derived from the host cell.

23.12 The major histocompatibility complex (MHC) in man:

1. is situated on chromosome 6
2. the genes are grouped into three types
3. is involved in antigen presentation
4. shows a positive association with Hodgkin's disease, multiple sclerosis and ankylosing spondylitis
5. is tested for by the laboratory on a serum sample

1. True

The MHC complex is located on the short arm of chromosome 6.

2. True

The genes have been grouped into three types, classes I, II and III.

3. True

MHC proteins play a crucial role in antigen presentation to T-cell receptors. Class I and II products provoke strong allograft rejection and have antigen-presenting functions. Class III products are components of the complement system.

4. True

Hodgkin's disease shows positive association with A1 and B8, multiple sclerosis with A3, B7 and DW2 and ankylosing spondylitis with B8.

5. False

MHC antigens are identified by the use of leucocyte suspensions. The term HLA is an abbreviation of the words human leucocyte antigen. Unclotted blood is needed by the laboratory.

23.13 Infection with HIV can cause:

1. an illness resembling acute glandular fever
2. persistent generalized lymphadenopathy
3. neurological complications
4. monoclonal B-cell activation
5. antibody formation within 7 days of exposure to infection

1. True

An illness resembling acute glandular fever occurs is some 10–20% of patients within a few weeks of infection and precedes seroconversion.

2. True

Persistent generalized lymphadenopathy occurs after a prolonged asymptomatic latent period and is followed by AIDS or ARC, (AIDS-related complex) in which lymphadenopathy, diarrhoea, night sweats, candidiasis and weight loss occur. Haematological examination reveals atypical lymphocytes and an increased number of CD8+ T cells.

3. True

These include acute aseptic meningitis, encephalopathy, myelopathy and neuropathy. Clinically, 70% of AIDS patients become demented.

4. False

In the later stages of infection, polyclonal B-cell activation occurs with an associated rise in the serum immunoglobulins, possibly due to direct activation of the B cells by the virus.

5. False

Antibody of HIV usually appears 3 weeks to 3 months after exposure and thereafter is detectable throughout the life of the patient. The antibodies are typically directed against the envelope glycoproteins.

23.14 The so-called 'Second Set' phenomenon:

1. occurs in an animal or human who has not previously rejected an allograft
2. occurs after a latent period of several days
3. depends on the graft antigenicity being recognised by the host T cells
4. can be demonstrated in both man and animals
5. can be delayed by prior irradiation of the graft

1. False
A 'Second Set' response only occurs in an animal or patient who has previously encountered an allograft.

2. False
A 'Second Set' response in a sensitised individual occurs within 2–3 days and in a highly sensitised individual, the graft may never become vascularized.

3. True
If the graft is unrecognised, as for example a graft placed in the anterior chamber of the eye, rejection will not occur.

4. True
A free allograft, e.g. skin, becomes vascularized in the same way as an isograft and remains viable for between 2–3 weeks, but in a Second Set response in a sensitised individual, graft rejection occurs within 2–3 days and the graft may never become vascularized at all.

5. True
Pretreatment of a graft by radiation reduces its immunogenicity, possibly by destroying highly immunogenic donor leucocytes of bone marrow origin.

23.15 Rejection of liver transplants is associated with:

1. arterial lesions
2. cholestasis
3. opportunistic infection
4. autoimmune chronic active hepatitis
5. multiple sclerosis

1. True
Arterial lesions develop in which a significant feature is the intimal accumulation of foamy lipid laden macrophages.

2. True
Canalicular cholestasis is present in chronic rejection, together with a destructive cholangitis and fibrotic changes in the protal tracts.

3. False
Opportunistic infections are not associated with rejection but with immunosuppression.

4. False
This appears to be inhibited by the immunosuppressive regime.

5. False
There is no association between liver transplantation and neurological disease.

23.16 Renal transplantation may be followed by:
1. infection
2. malignant neoplasia
3. amyloidosis
4. rheumatoid arthritis
5. psoriasis

1. True
However, it is not the transplant per se which predisposes to infection, but the suppression of immunity by the 'cocktail' of immunosuppressive drugs.

2. True
There is an increase in the incidence of squamous cell carcinoma of the skin and lymphoproliferative disorders. Many of these latter are Epstein Barr related.

3. False
Amyloidosis does not follow transplantation; it is associated with chronic infections.

4. False
Rheumatoid arthritis, an erosive arthropathy, is an autoimmune disease, possibly related to a viral infection.

5. False
Psoriasis is a skin disease of unknown aetiology. An increased incidence of the disease in certain HLA types suggests that genetic factors produce a predisposition to the development of the condition, but the basic cause has yet to be determined.

23.17 Acute rejection of a renal allograft involves:
1. cellular infiltration of the donor kidney
2. a humoral component
3. subacute vasculitis
4. polymorphonuclear infiltration of the graft
5. a fall in the serum creatinine

1. True
Acute rejection is accompanied by an extensive interstitial mononuclear infiltration of the kidney, consisting chiefly of medium and small-sized lymphocytes which immunoperoxidase staining reveals to be CD4+ and CD8+ lymphocytes.

2. True
The humoral element of acute rejection is manifested by a necrotising vasculitis which leads to extensive glomerular necrosis and cortical arteriolar thrombosis.

3. True
Subacute vasculitis is more common than necrotising vasculitis. The major finding is of a marked thickening of the renal arteries leading to luminal obstruction and a gradual failure of renal function.

4. False
Polymorphonuclear leucocytes play no part in the rejection phenomenon.

5. False
Evidence that rejection is occurring is shown by the rapid rise in the serum creatinine level.

23.18 HIV is:
1. a retrovirus
2. dependent on reverse transcriptase for its replication
3. causes a monoclonal hyperglobulininaemia
4. associated with the production of excessive amounts of IgG2
5. related to T-cell leukaemia

1. True
The human immunodeficiency virus, which is an enveloped RNA virus, has the capacity to make a DNA copy of itself through its characteristic enzyme, reverse transcriptase.

2. True
This enzyme reverses the normal process of gene replication and enables HIV to establish a latency similar to the DNA viruses, thus establishing a long term infection.

3. False
AIDS is associated with a polyclonal hypergammaglobulinaemia which results from the non-specific stimulation of B cells, predominantly causing the production of excessive amounts of IgG1, IgG3, IgA, IgD, IgE and in children, IgM.

4. False
Once AIDS has developed, the production of IgG2 is reduced. This is of particular importance in the defence against capsulated bacteria; this, together with a failure of B-cell response, accounts for the susceptibility of patients to bacterial infections.

5. True
Adult T-cell leukaemia has been shown to arise from infection with T-cell leukaemia virus Type 1 (NTLV1), a virus which causes unrestrained T-cell proliferation.

SECTION 24. MISCELLANEOUS

24.1 The following are referred to as 'Incomplete antibodies':
  1. IgD anti-D
  2. IgM anti-D
  3. anti-A isohaemagglutinin
  4. the Wassermann antibody
  5. tetanus antitoxin

1. True
IgG anti-D antibodies will not agglutinate D-positive erythrocytes in a saline solution alone. They require a colloid solution such as 30% bovine albumin or alternatively they can be detected by the use of the indirect Coombs test.

2. False
IgM anti-D antibodies will agglutinate D-positive erythrocytes in saline alone and they are, therefore, referred to as 'complete' antibodies. The terms 'complete' and 'incomplete' are used by haematologists to describe blood group antibodies only. The terms do not mean that structural deficiencies are present in the immunoglobulin molecule. Differences in reaction are probably a function of physical chemical forces.

3. False
Anti-A isohaemagglutinin is an IgM molecule and agglutinates blood group A erythrocytes directly in saline.

4. False
The Wassermann antibody is an IgM antibody which is present in individuals suffering from syphilis and other chronic infectious diseases. It is directed against an antigen present in cholesterolised extracts of bovine heart muscle, and is detected by a complement fixation test.

5. False
Tetanus antitoxin is demonstrated mainly by toxin neutralisation assay in mice. It can also be titrated by passive haemagglutination assay in which tetanus toxoid is bound to a red cell carrier.

24.2 The 'sick cell syndrome' is associated with:
  1. cardiac failure following surgery or trauma
  2. failure of the sodium pump
  3. a rise in the urinary sodium excretion
  4. apathy
  5. intracellular oedema

1. True
The 'sick cell syndrome' is specifically associated with operative intervention or trauma in patients who have suffered from cardiac failure over a prolonged period.

2. True
The underlying pathology of this syndrome appears to be a failure of the sodium pump at cell membranes throughout the body. The result is the passage of sodium into the intracellular space and the leakage of potassium.

3. False
Sodium excretion by the kidney diminishes but the excretion of potassium rises.

4. True
The classic clinical picture of the 'sick cell syndrome' is one of weakness and apathy developing on the third or fourth post-operative day. This is accompanied by a fall in the cardiac output, a poor peripheral circulation, bradycardia and a reduced digoxin tolerance.

5. True
The movement of sodium into the cells causes osmotic swelling to occur associated with the accumulation of water in the cytoplasm and separation of the organelles.

24.3 **The chief pathological and physiological changes in 'shock lung' include:**
1. intra-alveolar oedema and extravasation of erythrocytes into the alveoli
2. increased pulmonary compliance
3. infection
4. alkalosis
5. patchy opacities on the plain X-ray of the chest

1. True
Intra-alveolar oedema is the predominant change in the 'shock lung syndrome' and leads, if sufficiently severe, to respiratory failure. In addition erythrocyte extravasation occurs. The alveolar walls become lined with a hyaline membrane similar to that seen in hyaline membrane disease of the neonate. In the later stages if the patient survives, intra-alveolar fibrosis occurs.

2. False
Pulmonary compliance decreases in the 'shock lung' due to the combination of oedema and extravasation of erythrocytes. Because of this intermittent positive pressure ventilation may fail to produce any improvement in the oxygen tension.

3. True
Infection is a common complication of 'shock lung'. Bronchopneumonic change occurs adding an element of toxaemia to the general picture.

4. False
Acidosis accompanies the 'shock lung' and this may be irreversible despite therapy.

5. True

The typical radiological picture of a 'shock lung' is one of patchy opacities. These are attributed to a mixture of pulmonary oedema and collapse.

24.4 The compensatory mechanisms available to preserve the organism as a whole in the 'shock state' include:

1. autoregulation
2. a fall in the pO_2 of the blood
3. decreased pulmonary compliance
4. an increased sympatho-adrenal discharge
5. haemoconcentration

1. True

Autoregulation is the ability of an organ to maintain an adequate blood flow despite changes in the perfusion pressure. It is an intrinsic property of the smooth muscle of the blood vessels of the organ concerned and does not require the intervention of vasomotor nerves. Autoregulation occurs in the cerebral, coronary and renal vascular beds in which steady-state pressure-flow curves are seen until the systolic blood pressure is reduced to approximately 50 mmHg. Below this level a precipitous declino in blood flow follows.

2. False

A fall in the pO_2 does occur in severe shock but this is not a compensatory mechanism. The decrease in oxygen saturation of the systemic blood develops because oxygen has been extracted in such large amounts from the blood returning to the heart from the stagnating circulation. An additional factor in the later stages is the development of large right to left shunting.

3. False

Decreased compliance of the lungs may occur in severe shock but this is not a compensatory mechanism but a severe disadvantage to the shocked patient leading to the acute respiratory distress syndrome.

4. True

Increased sympatho-adrenal discharge results in increased myocardial contractility and constriction of the arterioles, both factors which tend to restore the blood pressure to normal levels. In addition, the added constriction of the capacitance vessels helps to maintain the venous return to the heart.

5. False

Increased blood viscosity occurs due to loss of the intravascular fluid but this is disadvantageous because it increases the resistance to blood flow particularly in the smaller blood vessels. Eventually widespread aggregation of red cells and platelets occurs, the sludging of blood, a phenomenon first described by Kniseley.

24.5   Which among the following are protozoal infections:
1. hydatid disease
2. trypanosomiasis
3. giardiasis
4. schistosomiasis
5. filariasis

1. False
Hydatid disease is caused by a cestode, (tapeworm) known as *Echinococcus granulosus* which is transmitted by dogs to man by faecal–oral contamination. The dog is infected by the eating of infected sheep, cattle or pig offal. Man ingests the ova which have a chitinous coat which is digested by the gastric juice thus liberating the embryos. These then invade the veins of the gastrointestinal tract and reach the liver via the portal blood, where most of them lodge to develop into unilocular or multilocular cysts.

2. True
The trypanosomes, *T. gambiense* and *rhodesiense* are both flagellated protozoa. Both are a cause of sleeping sickness, a disease transmitted by the tsetse fly. In South America another species, *T. cruzii*, which is transmitted by the blood sucking bugs of the family *Triatomidae*, causes a condition known as Chagas disease in which severe myocardial damage may occur.

3. True
Giardiasis is caused by the flagellate protozoa *Giardia lamblia*. This parasite causes an intestinal infection which leads to chronic diarrhoea and possible malabsorption.

4. False
Schistosomiasis is caused by a group of trematode worms which infect man after they have been released from their intermediate host. *Schistosoma haematobium* has as its intermediate host the snail, *Bulinus*, which lives in fresh but stagnant water. From the snail free swimming cercariae emerge which enter the human host chiefly through the skin of the legs and also through the mucous membrane of the mouth and pharynx. The adult worms finally reach the vesicle plexus of veins where they settle and pair. The major causes of damage are the ova which are produced. A granulomatous reaction is provoked with the result that fibrosis of bladder wall occurs. In addition squamous metaplasia of the urothelium may be followed by a squamous carcinoma. Another variety, the *Schistosoma mansoni*, inhabits the venules of the lower gastrointestinal tract provoking a granulomatous reaction with subsequent ulceration and melaena. Both may cause pipe-stem periportal fibrosis of the liver which may finally terminate in the development of portal hypertension and oesophageal varices.

5. False
Filariasis is a nematode infection, four different species of filaria can be found in human tissues. The diagnosis of filariasis is made by

demonstrating the presence of microfilariae in blood films at night in the case of *Wuchereria bancrofti* or in skin snip biopsies in the case of *Onchocerca volvulus*. Infestation with the former cause elephantiasis due to low grade inflammation which the parasite induces in the lymphatics and the latter causes subcutaneous nodules, looseness of the skin and blindness. *Wuchereria bancrofti* is transmitted by a female mosquito, usually of the *Culex* genus and onchocerca is transmitted by the fly, *Simulium damnosum*.

24.6 Mosquitoes transmit the following diseases:
1. schistosomiasis
2. leishmaniasis
3. dengue
4. yellow fever
5. malaria

1. False
The mosquito plays no part in the life cycle of the schistosoma, the intermediate host of this parasite is a snail found in fresh water, see 24.4.

2. False
Leishmaniasis is a protozoal disease transmitted by the bite of the sandfly, *Phlebotomus papatasi*. The condition is endemic throughout the Middle East, South Asia, Africa and Latin America. The infective agent is a slender, flagellated parasite which is introduced into the host together with the sandfly saliva. It is then phagocytosed by the mononuclear cells and transformed into a round amastigote which divides in the phagolysosomes of the macrophages, rupturing the cells and infecting others. The extent of the spread of the amastigotes is determined by the species of *Leishmania*. Thus the cutaneous form is caused by several varieties including *L. major* and *braziliensis* whereas visceral leishmaniasis is caused by *L. donovani* in the New World.

3. True
Dengue fever is a severe but usually short lived febrile illness which is caused by a toga virus transmitted by the mosquito *Aedes aegypti*.

4. True
Yellow fever is also caused by a toga virus transmitted by *Aedes aegypti*. Both the virus of dengue fever and yellow fever belong to the group collectively known as arthropod born virus, hence the generic name arbovirus.

5. True
Malaria is a protozoal disease transmitted by the female anopheles mosquito. The various protozoal species are *Plasmodium vivax*, *falciparum*, *malariae* and *ovale*. The most severe form of malaria is caused by *Pl. falciparum* which causes both cerebral malaria and

blackwater fever. The latter is so named because of the
haemoglobinuria which follows the severe intravascular haemolysis.

24.7   The following are mainly intracellular parasites:
1. *Echinococcus granulosus*
2. *Leishmania donovani*
3. *Trypanosoma gambiense*
4. *Plasmodium vivax*
5. *Toxoplasma gondii*

1. False
Echinococcus granulosus is a cestode (tapeworm) infestation which
gives rise to hydatid disease. The dog is the intermediate host
between sheep and man. In the latter the chief pathological lesion is
the formation of hydatid cysts. These are most commonly found in
the liver, lung, and brain, in descending order of frequency. The
worms themselves are extracellular and infection develops when ova
are accidently eaten. These are shed in the faeces of the dogs which
harbour the adult worm in the small intestine.

2. True
Leishmania donovani, a protozoon, is the causative agent of
systemic leishmaniasis, kala-azar, a disease in which the protozoa
are generally found within the macrophages in the amastigote form
called the Leishman–Donovan bodies. These are particularly common
in the bone marrow and spleen. Leishmania parasites are cleared
from the body by cell-mediated immune mechanisms. Hence the
diagnosis can be made by eliciting a delayed type of hypersensitivity
reaction to an extract of Leishmania injected into the skin, the
Leishmanin test.

3. False
The trypanosomes, *T. gambiense* and *T. rhodesiense* are flagellated
parasites which are found freely circulating in the blood. Both cause
sleeping sickness in cattle and the human and are transmitted from
man to man or from animals to man by the tsetse fly *(Glossina).*

4. True
Plasmodium vivax is one of a group of parasites of the genus
Plasmodium. This particular species is responsible for benign tertian
malaria. The diagnosis is confirmed by the examination of a blood
smear when various forms of the life cycle including trophozoites,
merozoites and schizonts can be seen within·infected erythrocytes.

5. True
Toxoplasma gondii, the cause of toxoplasmosis, multiplies within the
cytoplasm of the cells of the mononuclear phagocyte system causing
the lymph nodes to enlarge and become packed with large cells
which are probably macrophages. In severe cases cysts may form
and in the brain necrotic nodules may be found which may calcify.
Severe damage can also occur in the eye leading to choroidoretinitis

and uveitis. The definitive host is the cat and infection occurs through faecal contamination of the human either by inhalation or ingestion. In the cat oocysts are discharged into the lumen from their site of development in the gastrointestinal membrane.

24.8 Autosomal dominant diseases which are important to surgeons include:
1. hereditary spherocytosis
2. haemophilia
3. Von Recklinghausen's disease
4. familial agammaglobulinaemia
5. mucoviscidosis

1. True
Congenital spherocytosis (spherocytic haemolytic anaemia) is due to the erythrocytes being more nearly spherical than normal. The result is a condition in which the life span of the erythrocytes is reduced. The abnormal cells are sequestrated in the spleen. Clinically, anaemia, intermittent jaundice and increasing splenomegaly occur.

2. False
Although haemophilia is a disease of considerable surgical importance it is rare, affecting only 6 per 100 000 of the population. It is inherited as a sex–linked recessive Mendelian trait although sporadic cases do occur. It is transmitted to males by asymptomatic females who themselves possess a normal level of AHG of between 60–75% of the mean. Males with an AHG level of 25% of the mean can live a normal life but will bleed after major trauma, but when the level falls to between 1–5% minor trauma causes bleeding and haemoarthroses develop, these last occurring after very minor injuries when the level is less than 1%.

3. True
Von Recklinghausen's disease, otherwise known as neurofibromatosis, is associated with multiple nodules on the peripheral, and in some cases along the visceral branches of the sympathetic nerves. The disease is frequently associated with multiple pigmented patches of the skin, the café au lait spots. The various manifestations of this disease include:
  (a) Multiple subcutaneous nodules associated with café au lait spots
  (b) Dumb-bell tumours of the spinal nerves
  (c) Acoustic nerve neuroma
  (d) Elephantiasis neuromatosa
  (e) Plexiform neuromata

4. False
Otherwise known as infantile sex-linked hypogammaglobulinaemia this condition may exist in the presence of normal cell-mediated immunity. It is, however, inherited as an X-linked recessive. Affected

males have no B cells in their blood or lymphoid tissues and consequently their lymph nodes are small and they have no tonsils. IgA, IgM, IgD or IgE is not present in the serum. For the first 6 months of life, such infants are protected from infection by their maternal IgG which crossed the placenta. After this, in the absence of protection, the affected males develop recurrent pyogenic infections.

5. False
This condition is inherited as an autosomal recessive. To the surgeon this condition presents with congenital intestinal obstruction, the muscular power of the intestine being insufficient to propel the viscid meconium. To the paediatrician milder forms of the condition present with failure of the affected infant to thrive and recurrent pulmonary infections.

24.9 Chromosome abnormalities may occur:
1. in Klinefelter's syndrome
2. following treatment with methotrexate
3. as a result of ionising radiation
4. in Down's syndrome
5. in Christmas disease

1. True
This is one of the most frequent forms of genetic disease and hypogonadism involving the sex chromosomes. It occurs in approximately 1:850 live births. Its presence is rarely recognised before puberty, at which point the absence of testicular and penile enlargement becomes increasingly obvious. FSH levels are consistently elevated and the testosterone levels reduced.

2. False
Methotrexate does not directly affect the chromosomes.

3. True
Ionising radiation produces both 'sticky' chromosomes and breaks in the chromosomes, causing difficulties in the separation of the chromatids at anaphase.

4. True
Otherwise known as Trisomy 21, Down's syndrome is the commonest form of chromosomal disorder and a significant cause of mental retardation. In Trisomy 21, the extra chromosome results in a chromosome count of 47, although rarely the condition can arise from the translocation of chromosomal material leaving the chromosomal count at the normal figure of 46. The incidence of Down's is closely linked to maternal age, the condition occurring with increasing frequency with the advancing age of the mother, so that over 45 it affects 1:25 live births. This suggests that the primary fault lies in the ovum.

5. False
Christmas disease is clinically similar to haemophilia. It is not, however, associated with any chromosomal abnormality.

24.10 Serum levels of HBsAg may be high in:
1. lepromatous leprosy
2. tuberculosis
3. Down's syndrome
4. heroin addicts
5. malignant melanoma

1. True
The titre of HBsAg antigen tends to be high in the inmates of institutions such as prisons and leprosaria. Since the majority of individuals suffering from lepromatous leprosy are found in leprosaria, it follows that a higher than normal incidence of HBsAg positivity occurs in these patients.

2. False
Since the treatment of tuberculosis no longer requires long term residence in sanatoria an increased incidence of HBsAg positivity in this condition does not occur.

3. True
A higher incidence of HBsAg than normal has been reported in Down's syndrome. The cause for this remains unknown and is particularly difficult to explain since these patients are not usually confined to institutions or particularly immunodeficient.

4. True
Heroin addicts have a high incidence of HBsAg positivity because of their use of contaminated syringes and needles.

5. False
Patients suffering from neoplastic diseases do not appear to have an increased incidence of HBsAg positivity. They are, however, at risk if they require multiple transfusions or long stay residence in hospital.

24.11 The glycogen storage diseases are associated with the following enzyme defects:
1. amylase
2. glucose-6-phosphatase
3. amylo, 1, 6-glucosidase
4. glutamic oxaloacetic transaminase
5. nucleotide adenophosphodehydrogenase

1. False
Amylase is the enzyme secreted by the exocrine portion of the pancreas and is responsible for the digestion of carbohydrate. In

acute pancreatitis excessive quantities of this enzyme may be found in the blood enabling the diagnosis to be made.

2. True
Absence of this enzyme leads to von Gierke's disease (Type I glycogen storage disease). This disease develops in childhood and is associated with hepatomegaly and xanthomatosis.

3. True
A defect in this enzyme leads to a Type III glycogen storage disease, known eponymously as Ciris disease which resembles von Gierke's disease but is less severe.

4. False
Glutamic oxaloacetic transaminase is unrelated to glycogen storage diseases. It is an enzyme found in the liver, heart, kidneys and skeletal muscles concerned with transamination, i.e. the process whereby deamination of an amino acid is coupled with the amination of a ketoacid.

5. False
NADH dehydrogenase is an enzyme found in the brain. The energy status of any given area of the brain is most accurately expressed in terms of the ratio nucleotide adenophosphate (NAD^+) and NADH.

24.12 A vaccine:
1. contains one or more antigens
2. produces active immunity
3. contains one or more antibodies
4. stimulates polymorphonuclear leucocyte activity
5. can be administered orally

1. True
The aim of vaccine production is to alter a pathogen in such a way that it becomes harmless to the recipient but retains its antigenicity. Vaccines may be produced from bacteria or viruses and the organisms may be alive, attenuated or dead.

2. True
Active immunity is produced following the administration of a vaccine by the stimulation of antibody production by the plasma cells which are themselves derived from B lymphocytes.

3. False
Vaccines contain antigens. Immunisation against diphtheria toxin may be produced with toxin–antitoxin floccules (TAF).

4. False
A vaccine has no effect on polymorphonuclear leucocyte activity.

5. True
Vaccines may be administered in a number of ways. The most common orally administered vaccine is the poliomyelitis vaccine

introduced by Sabin which consists of living attenuated strains which have undergone mutation after passage through monkey-kidney cell cultures. The disadvantages associated with this type of vaccine are that the virus may not enter the cells of the intestinal tract and, therefore, no immunity develops and secondly, that the virus may undergo mutation in the alimentary tract reverting to a more virulent type which may then infect others.

24.13 Prostaglandins are:
1. formed from complement
2. vasodilators
3. involved in clotting
4. inhibited by azathioprine
5. inhibited by aspirin

1. False
Prostaglandins are derivatives of arachidonic acid which is released from mast cells and then metabolized by lipoxygenase or cycloxygenase enzymes depending on the type of mast cell to lipid metabolites, including PGD2. A further source of prostaglandins is the macrophage. Complement is an enzymatic system of serum proteins activated by antigen-antibody reactions.

2. True
Vasodilatation and increased capillary permeability are produced by PGE1 and PGE2, thus explaining the role of these compounds in acute inflammation. PGF2 protects the tissues from this action.

3. True
Prostaglandins are involved in clotting because a powerful platelet aggregator, thromboxane A2, is formed from prostaglandins G2 and H2. The enzymes involved are released when platelets become adherent to vessel walls.

4. False
Azathioprine does not inhibit the action of prostaglandins. It is, however, an immunosuppressive drug related to 6-mercaptopurine which is used in the treatment of diseases with an immunological basis including systemic lupus erythematosus, rheumatoid arthritis and Crohn's disease.

5. True
Aspirin inhibits the action of prostaglandins by the direct inhibition of their formation from the substrate arachidonic acid. This is thought to be the basis of its anti-inflammatory effect.